Ultrasound-Guided Percutaneous and Intraoperative Procedures

Guest Editor

WAEL E. SAAD, MBBCh, FSIR

ULTRASOUND CLINICS

www.ultrasound.theclinics.com

Consulting Editor
VIKRAM DOGRA, MD

July 2012 • Volume 7 • Number 3

SAUNDERS an imprint of ELSEVIER, Inc.

W.B. SAUNDERS COMPANY
A Division of Elsevier Inc.

1600 John F. Kennedy Boulevard • Suite 1800 • Philadelphia, Pennsylvania 19103-2899

http://www.theclinics.com

ULTRASOUND CLINICS Volume 7, Number 3
July 2012 ISSN 1556-858X, ISBN-13: 978-1-4557-3946-2

Editor: Donald Mumford

Ultrasound Clinics (ISSN 1556-858X) is published quarterly by W.B. Saunders, 360 Park Avenue South, New York, NY 10010-1710. Months of publication are January, April, July, and October. Business and editorial offices: 1600 John F. Kennedy Boulevard, Suite 1800, Philadelphia, Pennsylvania 19103-2899. Accounting and circulation offices: 6277 Sea Harbor Drive, Orlando, FL 32887-4800. Periodicals postage paid at New York, NY, and additional mailing offices. Subscription prices are $243 per year for (US individuals), $297 per year for (US institutions), $139 per year for (US students and residents), $273 per year for (Canadian individuals), $332 per year for (Canadian institutions), $291 per year for (international individuals), $332 per year for (international institutions), and $139 per year for (Canadian and foreign students/residents). To receive student/resident rate, orders must be accompanied by name of affiliated institution, date of term, and the signature of program/residency coordinator on institution letterhead. Orders will be billed at individual rate until proof of status is received. Foreign air speed delivery is included in all Clinics subscription prices. All prices are subject to change without notice. **POSTMASTER:** Send address changes to *Ultrasound Clinics,* Elsevier Health Sciences Division, Subscription Customer Service, 3251 Riverport Lane, Maryland Heights, MO 63043. **Customer Service (orders, claims, online, change of address): Telephone: 1-800-654-2452 (U.S. and Canada); 314-447-8871 (outside U.S. and Canada). Fax: 314-447-8029. E-mail: journalscustomerservice-usa@elsevier.com (for print support); journalsonlinesupport-usa@elsevier.com (for online support).**

Reprints: For copies of 100 or more, of articles in this publication, please contact the Commercial Reprints Department, Elsevier Inc., 360 Park Avenue South, New York, NY 10010-1710. Tel.: (+1) 212-633-3812; Fax: (+1) 212-462-1935; E-mail: reprints@elsevier.com.

Printed and bound by CPI Group (UK) Ltd, Croydon, CR0 4YY
Transferred to Digital Print 2012

Contributors

CONSULTING EDITOR

VIKRAM DOGRA, MD
Professor of Radiology, Urology, and
Biomedical Engineering, Director of Ultrasound
and Associate Chair for Education and
Research, Department of Imaging Sciences,
University of Rochester School of Medicine
and Dentistry, Rochester, New York

GUEST EDITOR

WAEL E. SAAD, MBBCh, FSIR
Professor of Radiology, Division of Vascular
Interventional Radiology , Department of
Radiology and Imaging, Sciences, University of
Virginia Health System, Charlottesville, Virginia

AUTHORS

MARYAM ASHRAF, MA
Graduate School of Arts & Sciences, University
of Virginia, Charlottesville, Virginia

MATTHEW R. BERNHARD, MD
Division of Vascular and Interventional
Radiology, Radiology and Medical Imaging,
University of Virginia Health System,
Charlottesville, Virginia

CHRISTIAN A. CHISHOLM, MD
Associate Professor, Department of Obstetrics
and Gynecology, The University of Virginia,
Charlottesville, Virginia

NIRVIKAR DAHIYA, MD
Assistant Professor, Section of Abdomen
Imaging, Mallinckrodt Institute of Radiology,
Washington University in St Louis, St Louis,
Missouri

GIA A. DEANGELIS, MD
Associate Professor of Radiology, University of
Virginia Health System, Charlottesville, Virginia

JAMES E. FERGUSON II, MD, MBA
Professor and Chair, Department of Obstetrics
and Gynecology, The University of Virginia,
Charlottesville, Virginia

MATTHEW R. GOSSAGE, MD
Radiology Resident, Department of Radiology
and Medical Imaging, University of Virginia,
Charlottesville, Virginia

JENNIFER A. HARVEY, MD
Professor of Radiology, Division Head-Breast
Imaging, University of Virginia Health System,
Charlottesville, Virginia

NICHOLAS J. HENDRICKS, MD
Radiology Resident, Department of Radiology,
University of Virginia, Charlottesville, Virginia

MINHAJ S. KHAJA, MD, MBA
Division of Vascular and Interventional
Radiology, Radiology and Medical Imaging,
University of Virginia Health System,
Charlottesville, Virginia

ALLISON J. LIPPERT, MD
Division of Vascular and Interventional
Radiology, Radiology and Medical Imaging,
University of Virginia Health System,
Charlottesville, Virginia

CHRISTINE O. MENIAS, MD
Professor, Section of Abdomen Imaging,
Mallinckrodt Institute of Radiology, Washington
University in St Louis, St Louis, Missouri

WILLIAM D. MIDDLETON, MD
Professor of Radiology, Section of Abdomen
Imaging, Mallinckrodt Institute of Radiology,
Washington University in St Louis, St Louis,
Missouri

HARUN OZER, MD
Department of Radiology, University of Virginia
Health System, Charlottesville, Virginia

WAEL E. SAAD, MBBCh, FSIR
Professor of Radiology, Division of Vascular
Interventional Radiology , Department of
Radiology and Imaging, Sciences,
University of Virginia Health System,
Charlottesville, Virginia

ROBERT F. SHORT, MD, PhD
Assistant Professor of Radiology, University
of Pittsburgh Medical Center, Pittsburgh,
Pennsylvania

PETER O. SIMON JR, MD
Resident Physician, Vascular and
Interventional Radiology / Special Procedures,
University of Virginia Health System,
Charlottesville, Virginia

ALECIA W. SIZEMORE, MD
Clinical Instructor, Radiology-Breast Imaging,
University of Virginia Health System,
Charlottesville, Virginia

JONATHAN K. WEST, MD
Division of Vascular and Interventional
Radiology, Radiology and Medical Imaging,
University of Virginia Health System,
Charlottesville, Virginia

Contents

> Ultrasound-guided vascular access is the initial step in an array of medical procedures. Ultrasound guidance has been shown to have numerous beneficial effects on accessing arterial and venous structures, including shortened procedure times, more precise access, and reduced morbidity/complication rates. This article discusses the indications, techniques, periprocedure management, imaging modalities, and outcomes related to ultrasound-guided vascular access.

> Pseudoaneurysm formation is a relatively common vascular complication of catheterization. Pseudoaneurysms can be a source of emboli, become infected, or rupture. This article sets out to review the indications, techniques, outcomes, and complications of the ultrasound guided pseudoaneurysm treatment. The most common treatment techniques for vascular access pseudoaneurysms are direct percutaneous thrombin injection and ultrasound-guided compression.

> Widely accepted as a minimally invasive, accurate, cost-effective technique, percutaneous image-guided biopsy has largely replaced diagnostic surgical biopsy in the evaluation of breast lesions. The natural curvature of the breast is used to advantage in ultrasound-guided breast interventions. Once mastered, free-hand technique is typically the fastest, most accurate method for ultrasound-guided procedures. Challenging cases require additional planning, however most breast lesions visible on ultrasound are amenable to ultrasound-guided biopsy. Contraindications and complications are few. This chapter focuses primarily on ultrasound-guided breast biopsy using freehand guidance. Many of these concepts can be transferred to other ultrasound-guided interventions.

> Amniocentesis and chorionic villus sampling are the most common techniques for obtaining a prenatal karyotype on a fetus at risk; in appropriately-trained hands, either can be performed with an acceptably low risk of complications. Ultrasound guidance is used for nearly all invasive diagnostic procedures in obstetrics, and seems to improve the odds for a successful procedure, but may not reduce the risk of procedure-related pregnancy loss. Ultrasound guidance is essential for fetal therapeutic interventions such as fetal blood transfusion, vesicoamniotic shunt placement, and thoracentesis.

allows more efficient PTC with or without percutaneous biliary drainage placement and helps avoid vascular injury. This article focuses primarily on US-guided left-sided bile duct access.

Percutaneous nephrostomy (PCN) is a procedure in which percutaneous access of the kidney is obtained to provide external drainage in an obstructed renal collecting system or serve as a conduit through which minimally invasive urologic procedures can be performed. Ultrasound-guided PCN has been validated as an effective and safe, minimally invasive image-guided procedure. This article reviews the indications, preprocedural patient evaluation, techniques, postprocedural management, and complications of ultrasound-guided PCN.

ULTRASOUND CLINICS

GOAL STATEMENT

The goal of the *Ultrasound Clinics* is to keep practicing radiologists and radiology residents up to date with current clinical practice in ultrasound by providing timely articles reviewing the state of the art in patient care.

ACCREDITATION

The *Ultrasound Clinics* is planned and implemented in accordance with the Essential Areas and Policies of the Accreditation Council for Continuing Medical Education (ACCME) through the joint sponsorship of the University of Virginia School of Medicine and Elsevier. The University of Virginia School of Medicine is accredited by the ACCME to provide continuing medical education for physicians.

The University of Virginia School of Medicine designates this enduring material activity for a maximum of 15 *AMA PRA Category 1 Credit*(s)™ for each issue, 60 credits per year. Physicians should claim only the credit commensurate with the extent of their participation in the activity.

The American Medical Association has determined that physicians not licensed in the US who participate in this CME enduring material activity are eligible for a maximum of 15 *AMA PRA Category 1 Credit*(s)™ for each issue, 60 credits per year.

Credit can be earned by reading the text material, taking the CME examination online at http://www.theclinics.com/home/cme, and completing the evaluation. After taking the test, you will be required to review any and all incorrect answers. Following completion of the test and evaluation, your credit will be awarded and you may print your certificate.

FACULTY DISCLOSURE/CONFLICT OF INTEREST

The University of Virginia School of Medicine, as an ACCME accredited provider, endorses and strives to comply with the Accreditation Council for Continuing Medical Education (ACCME) Standards of Commercial Support, Commonwealth of Virginia statutes, University of Virginia policies and procedures, and associated federal and private regulations and guidelines on the need for disclosure and monitoring of proprietary and financial interests that may affect the scientific integrity and balance of content delivered in continuing medical education activities under our auspices.

The University of Virginia School of Medicine requires that all CME activities accredited through this institution be developed independently and be scientifically rigorous, balanced and objective in the presentation/discussion of its content, theories and practices.

All authors/editors participating in an accredited CME activity are expected to disclose to the readers relevant financial relationships with commercial entities occurring within the past 12 months (such as grants or research support, employee, consultant, stock holder, member of speakers bureau, etc.). The University of Virginia School of Medicine will employ appropriate mechanisms to resolve potential conflicts of interest to maintain the standards of fair and balanced education to the reader. Questions about specific strategies can be directed to the Office of Continuing Medical Education, University of Virginia School of Medicine, Charlottesville, Virginia.

The faculty and staff of the University of Virginia Office of Continuing Medical Education have no financial affiliations to disclose.

The authors/editors listed below have identified no professional or financial affiliations for themselves or their spouse/partner:

Maryam Ashraf, MA; Matthew R. Bernhard, MD; Christian A. Chisholm, MD; Nirvikar Dahiya, MD; Gia A. DeAngelis, MD; James E. Ferguson II, MD, MBA; Matthew R. Gossage, MD; Jennifer A. Harvey, MD; Nicholas J. Hendricks, MD; Minhaj S. Khaja, MD, MBA; Allison J. Lippert, MD; Christine O. Menias, MD; William D. Middleton, MD; Donald Mumford, (Acquisitions Editor); Harun Ozer, MD; Peter O. Simon, Jr, MD; Robert F. Short, MD, PhD; Alecia W. Sizemore, MD; and Jonathan K. West, MD.

The authors/editors listed below have identified the following professional or financial affiliations for themselves or their spouse/partner:

Matthew J. Bassignani, MD (Test Author) is on the Advisory Board/Committee for Nuance and Fuji Medical Systems.
Vikram S. Dogra, MD (Consulting Editor) is the Editor of the Journal of Clinicl Imaging Science.
Wael E. Saad, MBBCh, FSIR (Guest Editor) is an industry supported research/investigator for Siemens, is a consultant for Boston Scientific, and is on the Speakers' Bureau for Atrium.

Disclosure of Discussion of Non-FDA Approved Uses for Pharmaceutical Products and/or Medical Devices

The University of Virginia School of Medicine, as an ACCME provider, requires that all faculty presenters identify and disclose any off-label uses for pharmaceutical and medical device products. The University of Virginia School of Medicine recommends that each physician fully review all the available data on new products or procedures prior to clinical use.

TO ENROLL

To enroll in the Ultrasound Clinics Continuing Medical Education program, call customer service at 1-800-654-2452 or visit us online at www.theclinics.com/home/cme. The CME program is available to subscribers for an additional fee of $196.00.

Preface

Ultrasound-Guided Percutaneous and Intraoperative Procedures

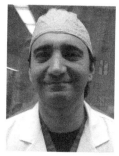

Wael E. Saad, MBBCh, FSIR
Guest Editor

Ultrasound is an invaluable modality for image-guided interventions. It is an extension of the operators' hand, providing real-time images irrespective of planes and without ionizing radiation. Moreover, Doppler ultrasound provides hemodynamic evaluation in vascular access cases and identifies vessels that are to be avoided in nonvascular access cases. As a result, ultrasound has permeated into numerous percutaneous and intraoperative minimally invasive procedures involving many body parts and organs.

This issue discusses the technical and clinical applications of ultrasound guidance of percutaneous and intraoperative image-guided minimally invasive procedures. It is written by volunteer authors and I am greatly indebted to their time commitment, devotion, and effort to this work.

Wael E. Saad, MBBCh, FSIR
Division of Vascular Interventional Radiology
Department of Radiology and Imaging Sciences
University of Virginia Health System
Charlottesville, VA, USA

E-mail address:
WS6R@virginia.edu

Ultrasound Clin 7 (2012) xi
doi:10.1016/j.cult.2012.04.002
1556-858X/12/$ – see front matter

Ultrasound-Guided Vascular Access

Peter O. Simon Jr, MD[a],*, Wael E. Saad, MBBCh, FSIR[b]

KEYWORDS

- Ultrasound-guided venous access • Ultrasound-guided arterial access
- Diagnostic ultrasonography • Hemostasis

KEY POINTS

- Ultrasound-guided vascular access is the initial step in an array of medical procedures.
- The adjunct of ultrasound guidance has been shown to have numerous beneficial effects on accessing arterial and venous structures, including shortened procedure times, more precise access, and reduced morbidity/complication rates.
- This article discusses the indications, techniques, periprocedure management, imaging modalities, and outcomes related to ultrasound-guided vascular access.

BROAD INDICATIONS

- Diagnostic angiography/venography
- Placement of indwelling reservoir/catheter/device
- Vascular access for the purpose of therapeutic intervention.

COMMON INDICATIONS FOR VENOUS ACCESS

Upper Extremity Veins

- Peripheral intravenous access for fluid, medication, or blood product infusions
- Venography
- Central venous access such as peripherally inserted central catheter (PICC) lines and reservoir devices (ports)
- Access for central venous interventions such as embolization procedures, venous thrombolysis, venoplasty, or stent placement
- Inferior vena cava (IVC)/superior vena cava (SVC) filter deployment.

Subclavian Vein

- Long-term central venous access for implants (temporary, tunneled, reservoir devices [ports], and cardiac devices)
- Access for central venous interventions such as pressure measurements, venous thrombolysis, venoplasty, or stent placement
- IVC/SVC filter deployment.

Internal Jugular Vein

- Long-term central venous access (tunneled, nontunneled, and reservoir devices [ports], and cardiac devices such as temporary pacers).
- Access for central venous interventions such as transjugular biopsy, transjugular intrahepatic portosystemic shunt placement (TIPS), pressure measurements, venous thrombolysis, venoplasty, or stent placement.
- IVC/SVC filter deployment
- Foreign-body retrieval
- Transvenous biopsies (such as renal, cardiac, liver)

[a] Vascular and Interventional Radiology / Special Procedures, University of Virginia Health System, 1215 Lee Street, PO Box 800170, Charlottesville, VA 22908, USA; [b] Division of Vascular Interventional Radiology, Department of Radiology and Imaging Sciences, University of Virginia Health System, Charlottesville, VA, USA
* Corresponding author.
E-mail address: peter.simon@virginia.edu

Ultrasound Clin 7 (2012) 283–297
doi:10.1016/j.cult.2012.04.001

- Reproductive therapies such as gonadal vein embolization.

Common Femoral Vein

- Access for central venous therapeutic interventions such as thrombolysis, venoplasty, stenting, or treatment of gastric varices (balloon-occluded retrograde transvenous obliteration)
- IVC/SVC filter deployment
- Secondary consideration for indwelling central venous catheters (tunneled catheters, nontunneled catheters, ports, and cardiac devices such as temporary pacers).
- Secondary consideration for indwelling central venous catheters (tunneled catheters, nontunneled catheters, ports, and cardiac devices such as temporary pacers)
- Secondary consideration for intrahepatic procedures
- Reproductive therapies such as gonadal vein embolization
- Adrenal vein or petrosal sinus sampling.

Below-the-Knee (Popliteal and Tibial) Veins

- Access for central venous therapeutic interventions
- Access for central venous interventions such as venous thrombolysis, venoplasty, or stent placement.

INDICATIONS FOR ARTERIAL ACCESS
Radial Artery

- Arterial pressure monitoring/blood gas analysis.

Brachial/Axillary Artery

- Aortography for diagnostic or therapeutic purposes
- Cardiac arteriography
- Cardiac catheterization (angioplasty/stent placement)
- Secondary site for abdominal or peripheral intervention such as angioplasty, stenting, stent-graft procedures or embolization
- Arterial pressure monitoring/blood gas analysis.

Carotid Artery

- Rarely used; may be considered in usual cases such as the treatment of an atypical aortic arch reconstruction or angioplasty procedure of the supra-aortic vessels.

Common Femoral Artery

- Access site of choice for most diagnostic and therapeutic catheter-based arterial interventions
- Angiography of virtually any vascular bed to include the mesenteric circulation, upper and lower extremity runoff, cardiac arteriography, carotid arteriography, and intracranial/intraspinal arteriography
- Intra-arterial therapeutic intervention to virtually any vascular bed to include embolization, angioplasty, stenting, stent-graft deployment, pressure measurement, therapeutic delivery of medication, arterial thrombolysis, and placement of indwelling intra-arterial devices.

VASCULAR ACCESS PRECAUTIONS AND PREPROCEDURAL EVALUATION

Guidelines for safe practices regarding coagulation status and hemostasis risk are outlined in **Table 1**. Each case whereby thresholds are exceeded must be evaluated individually, taking into account additional parameters such as patient's condition, surgical options, and resources available in an individual health system.

Initial Patient Evaluation

- Review previous cross-sectional imaging/laboratory studies.
- Evaluate for anomalous vessels.
- Evaluate vessel patency and course. For example, an occluded SVC would preclude an internal jugular vein approach for TIPS. Also, check for an enlarged inguinal hernia when planning a femoral vessel access.
- Evaluate for preexisting vascular injuries. Avoid access where there is a vascular injury from a prior access such as pseudoaneurysms, arteriovenous fistulas, and large hematomas.
- Obtain informed consent.
- Document a baseline vascular examination. The mainstay of the distal vascular examination is examination of the distal artery pulses (palpation, auscultation, Doppler ultrasonography), skin color, temperature, and capillary refill.
- A neurologic examination is required for carotid access or whenever the catheter reaches the aortic arch.

Preprocedural Imaging

Invasive diagnostic vascular evaluations have largely been replaced by noninvasive alternatives,

Table 1
Society of Interventional Radiology guidelines for coagulation status and hemostasis risk

Procedure	Bleeding Risk	Preprocedural Laboratory Studies	Management
Dialysis interventions	Low risk	INR, aPTT, Hct, Plt	INR >2.0: treatment with FFP or vitamin K
PICC line placement			Plt <50,000/μL: transfusion recommended
Venography			
IVC filter placement			
Arterial intervention up to 7F	Moderate risk	INR	INR >1.5: treatment with FFP or vitamin K
Venous intervention		aPTT (in setting of intravenous heparin use)	Plt <50,000/μL: transfusion recommended
Chemoembolization			Withhold clopidogrel for 5 days prior
Uterine fibroid embolization			
Tunneled central venous line			
Subcutaneous port device			
TIPS	Significant risk	INR, aPTT, Hct, Plt	INR >1.5: treatment with FFP or vitamin K
			Plt <50,000/μL: transfusion recommended
			Withhold clopidogrel for 5 days prior
			Withhold ASA for 5 days prior

Abbreviations: aPTT, activated partial thromboplastin time; ASA, acetylsalicylic acid; FFP, fresh frozen plasma; Hct, hematocrit; INR, international normalized ratio; IVC, inferior vena cava; PICC, peripherally inserted central catheter; Plt, platelet count; TIPS, transjugular intrahepatic portosystemic shunt.

Data from Malloy PC, Grassi CJ, Kundu S, et al. Consensus guidelines for periprocedural management of coagulation status and hemostasis risk in percutaneous image-guided interventions. J Vasc Interv Radiol 2009;20:S246–7.

which include cross-sectional imaging techniques such as computed tomography (CT) and magnetic resonance imaging. Review of any available images before undertaking an invasive intervention such as ultrasound-guided vascular access is crucial in selecting the most appropriate access route and avoiding vital structures, thus limiting potential complications.

General Procedural Risks for Ultrasound-Guided Vascular Access

- Hemorrhage
- Pain
- Neuropathy
- Pseudoaneurysms
- Dissection
- Arteriovenous fistula

- Infection to include cellulitis, abscess, fistula, and bloodstream infections with subsequent complications.

A current review of complication rates of femoral arterial ultrasound-guided vascular access is presented in **Table 2**. Complication rates of internal jugular and subclavian venous access with suggested thresholds is presented in **Table 3**. Finally, complication rates from upper extremity venous access are presented in **Table 4**.

Requisite Equipment

Ultrasound-related equipment

- Doppler-capable ultrasound machine
- Linear, high-frequency transducer (7.5 MHz or greater)

Table 2
Complications of ultrasound-guided femoral arterial puncture for diagnostic or therapeutic procedures

Complication	Incidence in FAUST Trial	Suggested Threshold Rate (%)
Hematoma ≥5 cm	0.6% (3/503)	2
Pseudoaneurysm	0.2% (1/503)	1
Dissection	0.4% (2/503)	1
Blood transfusion	0.2% (1/503)	1
Hematoma with DVT	0% (0/503)	1
Arteriovenous fistula	0% (0/503)	1
Any complication	1.4% (7/503)	<5

Abbreviations: DVT, deep venous thrombosis; FAUST, Femoral Arterial Access with Ultrasound Trial.

Data from Seto AH, Abu-Fadel MS, Sparling JM, et al. Real-time ultrasound guidance facilitates femoral arterial access and reduces vascular complications: FAUST (Femoral Arterial Access With Ultrasound Trial). JACC Cardiovasc Interv 2010;3(7):755.

- Sterile transducer cover
- Transducer guides are typically not necessary, although sometimes preferred by some practitioners.

Standard Surgical Preparation and Draping

- Chlorhexidine skin preparation solution

Table 3
Complications of internal jugular or subclavian venous access

Complication	Incidence (%)	Suggested Threshold Rate (%)
Pneumothorax	1–3	4
Hemothorax	1	2
Hematoma	1–3	4
Air embolus	1	2
Wound dehiscence	1	2
Procedure sepsis	1–3	4
Venous thrombosis	4	8

Data from Dariushnia SR, Wallace MJ, Siddiqi NH, et al. Quality improvement guidelines for central venous access. J Vasc Interv Radiol 2010;21:978.

Table 4
Complications of upper extremity venous access (PICCs and peripheral ports)

Complication	Incidence (%)	Suggested Threshold Rate (%)
Pneumothorax	0	0
Hemothorax	0	0
Arterial injury	0.5	1
Hematoma	1	2
Wound dehiscence	1	2
Procedure sepsis	1	2
Venous thrombosis	3	6
Phlebitis	4	8

Data from Dariushnia SR, Wallace MJ, Siddiqi NH, et al. Quality improvement guidelines for central venous access. J Vasc Interv Radiol 2010;21:978.

- Fenestrated drape or surgical drape material. Full body drape is considered standard, except under conditions whereby it is not practical (code situations, for example).

Local Anesthesia

- 21-gauge needle
- 1% lidocaine (with alternatives available in the event of patient allergy)
- Luer lock syringe.

Surgical Adjuncts

- 11-blade scalpel
- Sterile towels as necessary.

Graduated Access Devices

- Graduated, telescopic dilation system to initially gain access with 21-gauge needle (0.018-in wire) and to upsize to 0.035-in system. This system is typically referred to as a micropuncture kit and usually consists of a 2.5F to 3F inner dilator and a 4F to 5F outer dilator.
- Fascial dilator for the purpose of dilating a soft-tissue tract to allow a catheter/sheath to enter into a blood vessel with less resistance. The dilator is typically advanced over a 0.035-in guide wire.
- Peel-away sheath, used for the introduction of a tunneled central venous line or implantable port/reservoir catheter into a vascular territory.
- Side-port vascular sheath; used for maintaining a secure arterial or venous access for the purposes of exchanging diagnostic

catheters or interventional devices (typically 4F to 5F).

PROCEDURAL TECHNIQUE

For the purposes of this article, a general approach for ultrasound-guided vascular access is presented initially. Considerations specific to access site are then be addressed in subsequent sections.

Intravenous Access and Medication

- Intravenous access is necessary for the delivery of sedative medication and fluid resuscitation, and should be maintained until the patient is discharged. In selected cases (such as PICC line placement), the access to be placed may serve this purpose.

Preprocedure Ultrasonographic Evaluation

- Identify the target vessel and segment, typically done in the transverse plane to the target vessel. Be aware that some investigators and advance practitioners also advocate evaluation in the longitudinal plane to ensure targeting of the optimal segment and avoidance of adjacent structures.
- Perform mild compression to characterize adjacent vascular structures such as arteries and veins. Be aware that this examination can be confounded under conditions of elevated venous pressures (**Fig. 1**).
- Define a trajectory that avoids traversing structures that may be injured, such as adjacent arteries.
- It is important for the operator to consider not just puncturing the vessel, but rather entering the vessel at a favorable angle that allows for sufficient subcutaneous tissue coverage, avoids structures that may result in morbidity, and facilitates resistance-free advancement of the guide wire into the target vascular territory.
- During the planning scan, it is also useful to follow the course of the target vessel as much as possible, to identify any features that may preclude access such as a distal occlusive thrombus.

General Anatomic Considerations

- Under most conditions, arteries have a clearly discernible wall and veins have an imperceptible wall on high-frequency ultrasonography. During the initial evaluation, the provider should follow the target vessel distally as much possible to assess patency.
- Veins compress with less manual pressure than do arteries. Arteries are seen pulsating under manual compression when the adjacent vein is collapsed (see **Fig. 1**).
- Conditions under which veins are difficult to compress include thrombosis, large body habitus, profound edema, and extremity tenderness/lack of patient cooperation.

Standard Preparation of the Procedural Field

- Skin preparation in the target area is typically performed using chlorhexidine solution, achieved properly with a scrubbing motion. Existing protocols favor the use of 2 distinct, closely spaced cleansing episodes before draping the field.

A   **B**

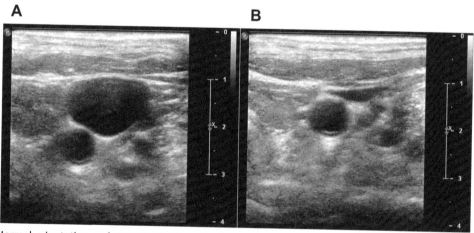

Fig. 1. Normal orientation and compressibility of the internal jugular vein. (A) Normal orientation of the internal jugular vein with respect to the carotid artery, with the vein maintaining a more superficial and lateral orientation. (B) Normal compressibility of the internal jugular vein.

- Place a fenestrated drape at the chosen and prepared skin region.
- Full body drape is considered standard, except under conditions whereby it is not practical (code situations, for example).

Local Anesthesia

- 1% lidocaine (or appropriate alternative) infiltration is performed using a 21-gauge or 23-gauge needle. A course should be chosen as a rehearsal to determine the optimal angle of needle entry.

VASCULAR TERRITORY–SPECIFIC FEATURES OF ULTRASOUND-GUIDED VASCULAR ACCESS

Ultrasound-Guided Vascular Access: Upper Extremity Veins

- Upper extremity veins are the most difficult to differentiate from adjacent arteries, this being particularly true in cases of low systemic pressures or in children. An emphasis should be placed on performing a careful preprocedure imaging evaluation.
- The ultrasound transducer is typically positioned transversely to the target vein and the 21-gauge beveled tip needle is advanced freely under ultrasound guidance.
- Adjusting the angle of the ultrasound transducer (often referred to as panning) allows the provider to observe the needle and needle tip as it is advanced to the desired target. The needle tip may then be observed indenting the superficial wall of the target arm vein inward toward the lumen, creating a concave surface. The needle tip has not entered the central lumen until the impaled superficial wall has rebounded and the needle tip is observed in the central lumen. A spontaneous return of blood may or may not be observed.
- At this point, a 0.018-in wire is carefully advanced through the needle, limiting movement of the needle itself.
- After the wire has been advanced carefully and without resistance, the remainder of the procedure is performed under fluoroscopic guidance.
- The guide wire is advanced carefully and without resistance under fluoroscopic guidance into the subclavian vein.
- After the wire has been advanced into the subclavian vein, a small (1–2 mm) incision is made using an 11-blade scalpel. The incision is performed over the needle body so as not to damage the guide wire.

- Next, a 4F to 5F transitional sheath is advanced over the wire while maintaining countertension on the guide wire (to prevent kinking of the guide wire).
- It is unnecessary to inject contrast agent to perform a venogram unless there is difficulty advancing the wire into the central veins.
- If venography is necessary, this is not typically performed via the access needle. Under such conditions, potential complications include losing vascular access and dissection. Instead, when necessary, venography is performed using a 2.5F to 3F micropuncture sheath that can be placed over the existing 0.018-in guide wire.
- Fig. 2 demonstrates the preprocedure and postprocedure ultrasonographic appearance of an upper extremity basilic vein PICC line placement.

Ultrasound-Guided Vascular Access: Subclavian Vein

- The subclavian vein is typically the most difficult to access by ultrasound because of the overlying bony structures that can limit visualization.
- The ideal target subclavian vein segment lies just over the lateral one-third of the first rib.
- If access is obtained in the medial segment, the catheter may pass through the scalene muscles and cause pain and constriction of the catheter with the motion of the patient's shoulder apparatus. This phenomenon has been referred to as pinch-off syndrome. Pinch-off syndrome often results in compression of the catheter, leading to poor flow. Over time, this process may fracture the catheter with the possibility of subsequent embolization of the catheter tip or extravasation of infused material.
- Adverse consequences of a far lateral placement include a higher risk of infection due to placement near the axilla, as well as unfavorable soft-tissue relationships if the generation of a catheter tunnel is desired.
- The ultrasound transducer is typically positioned transversely to the target segment of the subclavian vein, and the 21-gauge beveled tip needle is advanced freely under ultrasound guidance.
- Adjusting the angle of the ultrasound transducer (often referred to as panning) allows the provider to observe the needle and needle tip as it is advanced to the desired target. The needle tip may then be observed indenting the superficial wall of the

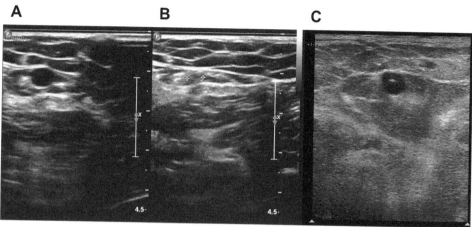

Fig. 2. Preprocedure and postprocedure appearance of the upper extremity basilic vein before and after peripherally inserted central catheter (PICC) line placement. (*A*) Normal gray-scale ultrasonographic appearance of the basilic vein. (*B*) Normal compressibility of a patent basilic vein. (*C*) Postprocedure appearance of the basilic vein after PICC line placement. The interval-placed catheter is clearly within the targeted vein without associated thrombus.

target vein inward toward the lumen, creating a concave surface. The needle tip has not entered the central lumen until the impaled superficial wall has rebounded and the needle tip is observed in the central lumen. A spontaneous return of blood may or not be observed.

- Unique to this approach, the needle may contact the surface of the first rib or clavicle. Particular attention should be directed to avoiding a pathway that crosses the pleural surface. It is this access approach that results in the highest incidence of pneumothorax.
- It is advised that this vessel be aspirated before the placement of the 0.018-in guide wire. Because of a close relationship with the subclavian artery and the inability to compress the vessel beneath the rib cage, an inadvertent arterial puncture is possible. Under most conditions, the puncture needle may be withdrawn and the patient can be observed for complications before reattempts at access.
- At this point, a 0.018-in wire is carefully advanced through the needle, limiting movement of the needle itself.
- After the wire has been advanced carefully and without resistance, the remainder of the procedure is performed under fluoroscopic guidance.
- Several attempts may be necessary to advance the guide wire into the SVC. The ability to access the SVC may be affected by the curve at the tip of the wire as well as the patient's phase on respiration. Under

circumstances when the 0.018-in wire does not immediately course toward the SVC, rotating the guide wire as well as advancing the wire during deep inspiration may affect successful placement into the SVC.

- After the wire has been advanced into the SVC, a small (1–2 mm) incision is made using an 11-blade scalpel. The incision is performed over the needle body so as not to damage the guide wire.
- Next, a 4F to 5F transitional sheath is advanced over the wire while maintaining countertension on the guide wire (to prevent kinking of the guide wire). This action is typically followed by the placement of a more robust wire such as a 0.035-in guide wire.
- A venogram is not routinely performed except under conditions whereby there is difficulty advancing the guide wire into the SVC.
- Postaccess imaging is typically obtained (either by fluoroscopic spot film or formal chest radiograph), as this site carries a higher risk for pneumothorax. If a pneumothorax is not detected but the patient develops respiratory symptoms in the recovery area, the patient should be evaluated and repeat imaging should be promptly performed.

Ultrasound-Guided Vascular Access: Internal Jugular Vein

- The ultrasound transducer is typically positioned transversely to the internal jugular vein and the 21-gauge beveled tip needle is advanced freely under ultrasound guidance.

- Adjusting the angle of the ultrasound transducer (often referred to as panning) allows the provider to observe the needle and needle tip as it is advanced to the desired target. The needle tip may then be observed indenting the superficial wall of the target vein inward toward the lumen, creating a concave surface. The needle tip has not entered the central lumen until the impaled superficial wall has rebounded and the needle tip is observed in the central lumen.
- Some operators choose to alternatively access the vein with the transducer placed transversely to the vessel, but the needle inserted along the long access of the transducer, approaching from the lateral plane. This technique is favored by some practitioners for the purposes of placing a tunneled line, especially in obese patients. This approach may facilitate passing the needle access as close to the clavicle as possible, which allows for the formation of a smooth curve and limited movement of the catheter when the patient's soft tissues change position (when elevated from supine back to upright). An adverse consequence of this approach is the tendency for the wire to migrate in the cranial direction.
- At this point, a 0.018-in wire is carefully advanced through the needle, limiting movement of the needle itself. If it is not clear by ultrasonography that the vessel has been entered, aspiration of the needle can be performed. The potential downside to this maneuver is the additional movement may cause dislodgment of the needle from the vessel.

- After the wire has been advanced carefully and without resistance, the remainder of the procedure is performed under fluoroscopic guidance.
- After the wire has been advanced into the SVC, a small (1–2 mm) incision is made using an 11-blade scalpel. The incision is performed over the needle body so as not to damage the guide wire.
- Next, a 4F to 5F transitional sheath is advanced over the wire while maintaining countertension on the guide wire (to prevent kinking of the guide wire). This action is typically followed by the placement of a more robust wire such as a 0.035-in guide wire.
- After the transition has been completed, preparations can be made for catheter placement such as tunnel generation and/or peel-away sheath placement.
- **Fig. 3** demonstrates the typical sequence of maneuvers performed during access of the internal jugular vein using ultrasonography. The maneuvers shown here form the basis for obtaining vascular access at other anatomic locations.

Ultrasound-Guided Vascular Access: Femoral Vein

- Fluoroscopy is used for the purposes of localizing the mid-segment of the femoral head. This site is chosen because it allows for manual compression of the vessel against this structure to obtain hemostasis. This site also provides a favorable relationship, as the femoral artery and vein are adjacent to one another in the transverse plane at this level (**Figs. 4** and **5**).
- Another consideration when evaluating the vessel during preoperative ultrasonography

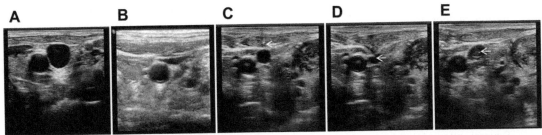

Fig. 3. Ultrasonographic appearance of the internal jugular vein during puncture. (*A*) Normal orientation of the carotid artery and internal jugular vein. (*B*) Typical compressible nature of the more lateral internal jugular vein. In (*C*) the arrow marks the appearance of the access needle as it is directed toward the internal jugular vein. In (*D*) the access needle is seen "tenting" the internal jugular vein, just before entry (*arrow*). In (*E*) the successful puncture with the needle tip within the center of the vein lumen is indicated (*arrow*).

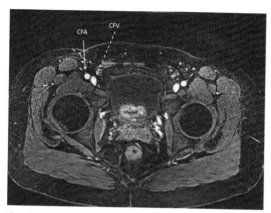

Fig. 4. Normal anatomic relationships of the femoral vessels. Contrast-enhanced magnetic resonance imaging through the pelvis displays the normal anatomic relationships of the common femoral artery (CFA) and common femoral vein (CFV) at the level of the femoral head.

is the relationship of the profunda femoris. If fluoroscopy is unavailable, a useful ultrasound landmark is the common femoral vein caudal to its bifurcation.

- The ultrasound transducer is typically positioned transversely to the common femoral vein, and the 21-gauge beveled tip needle is advanced freely under ultrasound guidance.

- Adjusting the angle of the ultrasound transducer (often referred to as panning) allows the provider to observe the needle and needle tip as it is advanced to the desired target. The needle tip may then be observed indenting the superficial wall of the target vein inward toward the lumen, creating a concave surface. The needle tip has not entered the central lumen until the impaled superficial wall has rebounded and the needle tip is observed in the central lumen.

- The angle of entry is important for the introduction of therapeutic devices or large sheaths. Any angle too steep may result in kinking of an introducer sheath and should be avoided.

- Once the vein has been entered, a 0.018-in guide wire is carefully advanced through the needle, limiting movement of the needle itself. If it is not clear by ultrasonography that the vessel has been entered, aspiration of the needle can be performed. The potential downside to this maneuver is the additional movement may cause dislodgment of the needle from the vessel.

- After the wire has been advanced carefully and without resistance, the remainder of

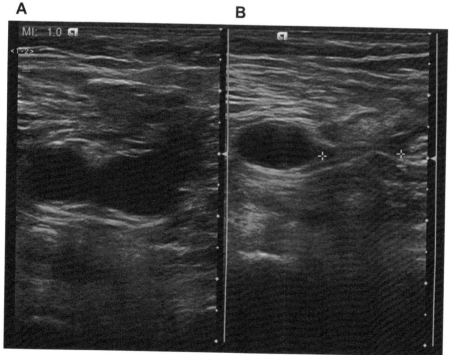

Fig. 5. Ultrasonographic appearance of the common femoral vessels. (*A*) Normal ultrasonographic appearance of the common femoral artery and vein. (*B*) The compressible nature of the common femoral vein is evident, allowing for clear identification for the purposes of planning vascular access. Calipers represent the compressed medial and lateral margins of the common femoral vein.

the procedure is performed under fluoroscopic guidance.

- After the wire has been advanced into the IVC, a small (1–2 mm) incision is made using an 11-blade scalpel. The incision is performed over the needle body so as not to damage the guide wire. Under most circumstances, the IVC lies to the right of the spine.
- Next, a 4F to 5F transitional sheath is advanced over the wire while maintaining countertension on the guide wire (to prevent kinking of the guide wire). This action is typically followed by the placement of a more robust wire such as a 0.035-in guide wire.
- A venogram is not routinely performed except under conditions whereby there is difficulty advancing the guide wire into the IVC.
- After the transition has been completed, preparations can be made for catheter or device placement.

Ultrasound-Guided Vascular Access: Lower Extremity Veins (Popliteal or Tibial Veins)

- Lower extremity veins are infrequently accessed. If access is necessary, this is most frequently for the treatment of acute or chronic deep venous thrombosis, often for the purposes of venous thrombolysis. Additional interventions after thrombolysis may include therapy for an outflow stenosis or chronic thrombus using balloon venoplasty followed by stent placement.
- The ultrasound transducer is typically positioned transversely to the target vein, and the 21-gauge beveled tip needle is advanced freely under ultrasound guidance.
- Adjusting the angle of the ultrasound transducer (often referred to as panning) allows the provider to observe the needle and needle tip as it is advanced to the desired target. The needle tip may then be observed indenting the superficial wall of the target vein inward toward the lumen, creating a concave surface. The needle tip has not entered the central lumen until the impaled superficial wall has rebounded and the needle tip is observed in the central lumen.
- For interventions such as thrombectomy/ thrombolysis, large vascular sheaths are typically necessary. In addition, because these sheaths are commonly indwelling for periods of 24 to 72 hours, an obtuse (rather than steep) angle is favored. Such planning of skin and vessel entry sites can limit the

incidence of kinking of the vascular sheath after insertion.

- Once the vein has been entered, a 0.018-in guide wire is carefully advanced through the needle, limiting movement of the needle itself. If it is not clear by ultrasonography that the vessel has been entered, aspiration of the needle can be performed. The potential downside to this maneuver is the additional movement may cause dislodgment of the needle from the vessel.
- After the wire has been advanced carefully and without resistance, the remainder of the procedure is performed under fluoroscopic guidance.
- After the wire has been advanced more centrally, a small (1–2 mm) incision is made using an 11-blade scalpel. The incision is performed over the needle body so as not to damage the guide wire.
- Next, a 4F to 5F transitional sheath is advanced over the wire while maintaining countertension on the guide wire (to prevent kinking of the guide wire). This action is typically followed by the placement of a more robust wire such as a 0.035-in guide wire.
- At this point, a venogram is routinely performed to evaluate the extent of existing thrombus and to characterize the venous access/vascular territory.

Ultrasound-Guided Vascular Access: Upper Extremity (Radial, Brachial, and Axillary) Arteries

- Upper extremity arteries are the most difficult to differentiate from adjacent veins, and this is particularly true in cases of low systemic pressures or in children. An emphasis should be placed on performing a careful preprocedure imaging evaluation.
- The ultrasound transducer is typically positioned transversely to the target artery, and the 21-gauge beveled tip needle is advanced freely under ultrasound guidance.
- Adjusting the angle of the ultrasound transducer (often referred to as panning) allows the provider to observe the needle and needle tip as it is advanced to the desired target.
- On entry into the arterial lumen, pulsatile blood return typically occurs.
- Once the artery has been entered, a 0.018-in guide wire is carefully advanced through the needle, limiting movement of the needle itself.

- After the wire has been advanced carefully and without resistance into the artery, the remainder of the procedure is performed under fluoroscopic guidance.
- After the wire has been advanced into the subclavian artery, a small (1–2 mm) incision is made using an 11-blade scalpel. The incision is performed over the needle body so as not to damage the guide wire. The incision should also be superficial as not to damage the underlying artery.
- Next, a 4F to 5F transitional sheath is advanced over the wire while maintaining countertension on the guide wire (to prevent kinking of the guide wire). This action is typically followed by the placement of a more robust wire such as a 0.035-in guide wire.
- After the transition has been completed, preparations can be made for subsequent diagnostic or therapeutic intervention.
- **Fig. 6** demonstrates imaging features that allow for differentiation of the brachial artery and veins.

Ultrasound-Guided Vascular Access: Common Femoral Artery

- The typical cross-sectional and ultrasonographic appearance of the common femoral vessels are demonstrated in **Figs. 4** and **5**.
- Entry into the femoral artery at the level of the mid-portion of the femoral head is desired, because of the ability to compress the vessel against the bony landmark after catheter removal as well as its favorable orientation (side-to-side) with the femoral vein.
- The site of entry into the vessel is estimated using a metallic marker and fluoroscopy, and a skin mark is made. After the desired arterial entry site is selected, the ultrasound probe is placed transversely over the vessel

and a skin entry site is selected that will allow the needle to enter the skin and artery at an approximate 45° angle (entering the vessel at the level of the mid-portion of the femoral head).
- Using ultrasound guidance, a 21-gauge or 18-gauge beveled tip needle is typically advanced into the artery using a single-wall technique (puncturing the superficial wall and then advancing the wire through the needle).
- Adjusting the angle of the ultrasound transducer (often referred to as panning) allows the provider to observe the needle and needle tip as it is advanced to the desired target.
- On entry into the arterial lumen, pulsatile blood return typically occurs.
- Once the artery has been entered, an appropriately sized guide wire is carefully advanced through the needle, limiting movement of the needle itself.
- After the wire has been advanced carefully and without resistance into the artery, the remainder of the procedure is performed under fluoroscopic guidance.
- An alternative technique is referred to as the double-wall method. This approach is unique in that the puncture needle is advanced through both the superficial and deep walls of the artery until it contacts the femoral head. After the needle has contacted the femoral head, the wire can be safely handled with the opposite hand and the needle can be carefully withdrawn, and the guide wire inserted after blood return is seen. The primary advantage to this approach is that the ultrasound transducer is not needed after initial vessel puncture and can therefore be placed away from the field, freeing an extra hand for additional stability.

A **B** **C**

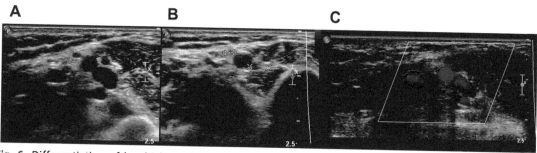

Fig. 6. Differentiation of brachial arteries and veins. (*A*) Typical ultrasonographic appearance of the brachial vessels, superficial to the humerus. (*B*) The compressibility of the brachial veins is seen, allowing the brachial artery to be clearly differentiated. In cases where compression is difficult to achieve, color Doppler (*C*) is a useful adjunct, allowing for the differentiation of the brachial vessels based on differential direction of blood flow.

- Once the wire has been advanced, an incision is made using an 11-blade scalpel at a depth of 3 mm. The blade incision is made over the needle so as not to damage the wire.
- A 4F to 5F transitional sheath (micropuncture dilator) is passed over the wire while holding countertension on the wire so as not to kink the wire, thus allowing the operator to pass a more robust wire.
- A side-port sheath is then placed and flush lines are connected in standard fashion.
- **Fig. 7** shows the ideal imaging features of appropriate placement in the femoral artery. Of note, puncture of the vessel is performed below the level of the inguinal ligament in most cases.

SITE-SPECIFIC POSTACCESS HEMOSTASIS
Venous Access Sites

- Manual compression for 5 minutes is performed except under conditions of

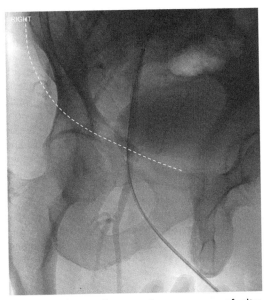

Fig. 7. Satisfactory fluoroscopic appearance of ultrasound-guided arterial sheath placement. This single fluoroscopic image taken after hand injection of intra-arterial contrast agent through the side port of a vascular sheath placed using ultrasound guidance shows the ideal imaging features of appropriate placement in the femoral artery. Specifically, the common femoral artery is entered at the mid-portion of the femoral head, allowing for compression against this structure to control hemorrhage. The bifurcation of the profunda femoris is also clearly seen, anatomically allowing for the deployment of a vascular closure device, if clinically indicated. The dashed line represents the approximate anatomic course of the inguinal ligament.

coagulopathy or distal venous obstruction, which may require longer periods of manual compression.
- Bleeding risk at the internal jugular site can be increased by coughing.
- Purse-string sutures may be used in select circumstances to control bleeding from venous access sites, but should be used with caution.

Axillary Artery Access Site

- Manual pressure can be exerted on the axillary artery access site. Manual pressure is maintained while the arm is in mid-abduction and is exerted against the humeral head for a period of 10 to 15 minutes in the absence of coagulopathy.
- The arm should be maintained overnight in a sling to support a neutral position. Distal pulses should be monitored and referenced with the initial baseline pulse examination.

Femoral Artery Access Site

- Manual pressure is maintained on the femoral artery access site to obtain hemostasis. Manual pressure is adjusted to occlude the access site, but not enough to occlude the femoral artery and compromise distal flow. A Doppler probe is a useful adjunct for monitoring of the artery and estimating the degree of manual pressure required.
- Manual pressure is maintained with the patient in a supine position. Manual pressure is maintained against the underlying femoral head for a period of 15 to 20 minutes in the absence of coagulopathy. A useful guideline is 3 minutes of manual compression for each 1F size of the access device.
- A thorough pulse examination before, during, and after access/hemostasis is crucial for the purposes of identifying changes (such as thrombosis/embolic phenomena).
- Numerous percutaneous closure devices are available, which reduce the period of manual compression necessary to achieve hemostasis and reduce the bed-rest period, thus allowing earlier discharge of the patient. Refer to the product insert for device-specific recommendations.
- At the authors' institution and in the absence of a closure device, for the purposes of diagnostic arteriography, the patient must be flat for 2 hours and then may have the head elevated for an additional 2 hours, after

which ambulation is permitted. When an intervention is performed, the head may be elevated at 6 hours, and the patient is on strict bed rest until the next morning.

POST-ACCESS PROCEDURAL EVALUATION AND MANAGEMENT
Postprocedural Observation Period

- In the absence of conscious sedation, patients receiving a basic venous access procedure such as a PICC line may be discharged immediately.
- When sedative medications are used, patients undergoing tunneled line placement, port placement, or IVC filter removal may be discharged to the care of a responsible adult within 1 hour of full recovery from sedative medication.
- In cases when more extensive procedures are performed, patients are typically observed overnight in the hospital. Ultimately, the length of stay is determined by the patient's existing medical problems and the most extensive portion of the procedure.
- Patients undergoing diagnostic arterial angiography may be discharged 6 to 8 hours after the procedure in the absence of a closure device. With the use of an arterial closure device this period can be reduced to 4 hours.
- In the case of femoral arterial puncture, the patient should not travel by car (hip flexed) for longer than 1 hour on the day of the procedure.

Managment of Fluids, Diet, and Activity

- Intravenous access should be maintained until the patient is ready for discharge.
- After the patient has recovered from sedation (if administered), a clear liquid diet should be tolerated before discharge.
- Intravenous fluids, in the appropriate clinical setting, should be administered until the patient has tolerated a clear liquid diet.
- At the authors' institution, for PICC lines and venography performed with peripheral intravenous access, the patient may ambulate immediately. For more advanced diagnostic and therapeutic venous procedures the head may be elevated immediately, but the patient must remain on bed rest for 2 hours.
- In the event the patient coughs, sneezes, strains, or laughs, the patient must apply manual pressure to the puncture site.

- At the authors' institution, patients undergoing diagnostic arteriography and treated with a closure device may have the head elevated to 30° immediately, with ambulation at 2 hours and discharge at 4 hours. In the absence of a closure device, patients must lie flat for 2 hours and may ambulate at 4 hours. Patients undergoing therapeutic arterial interventions without a closure device may elevate the head of the bed at 6 hours and are maintained on strict bed rest overnight.
- For closure devices, refer to device-specific instructions for further details.
- The accessed extremity is maintained straight for the bed-rest period.
- Strict bed rest includes no bathroom privileges. In these cases, the patient must use a bedpan or other method of collection.

Analgesia and Medications

- Pain after routine ultrasound-guided vascular access is typically minimal and is classified as mild to moderate (for the first 24 hours). More severe pain should raise suspicion for a complication, and warrants direct evaluation.
- In the setting of tunnel or port placement, a patient may require short-term narcotic pain medication for control of analgesia. Combinations of acetaminophen and hydrocodone are commonly used for this purpose. Intravenous analgesic medication is uncommon for the purpose of routine ultrasound-guided vascular access.
- When the vascular access is performed as part of a more extensive procedure such as embolization of a mass (eg, uterine fibroid embolization), patients may require intravenous narcotic medications for adequate treatment of analgesia. Commonly used analgesics include fentanyl, morphine, or hydromorphone patient-controlled analgesia, commonly used for 12 to 48 hours depending on the nature of the procedure and the patient.
- Antiemetics such as ondansetron may be helpful in the setting of embolization procedures, conscious sedation, or in the event of an adverse reaction resulting in nausea.
- For the sole purposes of ultrasound-guided vascular access, systemic antibiotics are typically unnecessary. The use of antibiotics is typically determined by the main procedure performed (port implantation, embolization, and so forth).

- For the purposes of routine vascular access, home prescription–strength analgesic medications are typically not prescribed. If the vascular access is performed as part of a more extensive procedure, that portion dictates the need for discharge analgesic medications.

Post Procedure Monitoring

- Routine monitoring should include heart rate, blood pressure, and oxygen saturation.
- These parameters should occur at 15-minute intervals.
- In the setting of conscious sedation, labile blood pressure should be anticipated, which may be due to vasodilatory effects of medication, hypovolemia, or hemorrhage. Initial therapy should include volume resuscitation and a heightened awareness, warranting intervention if the patient does not respond appropriately.
- If the patient does not respond appropriately, a source of hemodynamic instability should be sought and appropriate resuscitative measures should be initiated. Appropriate management is addressed below. Imaging evaluation often is performed using CT.
- Particularly in the case of arterial interventions, a baseline vascular examination is essential in monitoring the success of a procedure as well as complications. A change in pulse can alert the practitioner to the presence of emboli, compressive hematoma, or dissection.
- In the case of aortic arch or cerebrovascular circulation, a baseline neurologic examination is useful in detecting stroke.

COMPLICATIONS AND MANAGEMENT
Management of Postprocedure Hemorrhage

- Intravenous access should be maintained until the patient is ready for discharge in the event that fluid resuscitation or intravenous medication is required.
- Several types of postprocedure hemorrhage may occur:
  - Skin hemorrhage
  - Target-vessel hemorrhage
  - Site hematomas (which may result in a secondary neuropathy in the case of upper arterial punctures)
  - Retroperitoneal hematoma
  - Hemothorax.

- Management of significant bleeding should be initially managed by maintaining adequate vascular access, obtaining a type, cross and coagulation parameters (prothrombin time, international normalized ratio, partial thromboplastin time), cessation or reversal of anticoagulation (such as heparin), and administering isotonic resuscitation fluid. Further management may include critical care or surgical consultation.
- In the setting of active hemorrhage, blood transfusion should be considered to maintain a hematocrit greater than 30%. Guidelines for higher transfusion thresholds are not intended for the actively hemorrhaging patient.
- Imaging evaluation may include chest radiograph to evaluate for hemothorax and noncontrast CT to evaluate for retroperitoneal bleeding.

Management of Thoracic Complications

- If postprocedure chest pain occurs, chest radiography should be performed to evaluate for pneumothorax or hemothorax.
- Clinically meaningful pneumothorax or hemothorax is typically treated with a thoracostomy tube, supplemental oxygenation, and resuscitation (in the case of hemothorax).
- If a small, asymptomatic pneumothorax occurs, tube thoracostomy may not be required. Repeat imaging is performed in 1 hour. A thoracostomy tube is indicated if the patient is symptomatic or there is expansion of the pneumothorax.

Management of Infectious Complications

- Abscess at the vascular access site, like abscesses elsewhere, are treated with surgery.
- Local infections related to implants, such as catheters and ports, should prompt removal of the foreign body with possible open drainage of the access site.
- Broad-spectrum antibiotics that cover the likely offending organism may be used, narrowed to appropriate culture results.

Management of Vascular Injuries

- Include arterial dissection, arteriovenous fistula, or pseudoaneurysms.
- Dissection should be identified at the time of the procedure. In the event of a flow-limiting injury, a stent should be deployed. If the injury is not flow limiting, observation with imaging follow-up with or without anticoagulation is a treatment option.

- Arteriovenous fistulas are rarely recognized during the inciting procedure. Such an injury typically is noted on follow-up clinical or imaging examination. The initial treatment of choice for a physiologically meaningful fistula is endovascular therapy. Surgical consultation may be necessary in some cases.
- Pseudoaneurysms are often treated with thrombin injection.

FURTHER READINGS

Dariushnia SR, Wallace MJ, Siddiqi NH, et al. Quality improvement guidelines for central venous access. J Vasc Interv Radiol 2010;21:976–81.

Denys BG, Uretsky BF, Reddy PS, et al. An ultrasound method for safe and rapid central venous access. N Engl J Med 1991;324(8):566.

Dogra V, Saad WE. Ultrasound-guided procedures. New Yark: Thieme Medical Publisher; 2009.

Malloy PC, Grassi CJ, Kundu S, et al. Consensus guidelines for periprocedural management of coagulation status and hemostasis risk in percutaneous image-guided interventions. J Vasc Interv Radiol 2009;20: S240–9.

Seto AH, Abu-Fadel MS, Sparling JM, et al. Real-time ultrasound guidance facilitates femoral arterial access and reduces vascular complications: FAUST (Femoral Arterial Access With Ultrasound Trial). JACC Cardiovasc Interv 2010;3(7):751–8.

Ultrasound-Guided Management of Vascular Access Pseudoaneurysms

Nicholas J. Hendricks, MD[a],*, Wael E. Saad, MBBCh, FSIR[b]

KEYWORDS

- Pseudoaneurysm • Ultrasound-guided management • Percutaneous thrombin injection
- Compression

KEY POINTS

- Pseudoaneurysms can be a source of emboli, become infected, or rupture.
- The most common treatment techniques for vascular access pseudoaneurysms are direct percutaneous thrombin injection and ultrasound-guided compression.
- The most common complication of pseudoaneurysm compression is procedural pain.
- Distal arterial embolization is the most common and worrisome adverse effect of direct percutaneous thrombin injection.

INTRODUCTION

Pseudoaneurysm formation is a relatively common vascular complication of catheterization. They develop because of a disturbance in the arterial wall, which forms a profused outpouching contained by media, adventitia, or surrounding soft tissues. This pseudoaneurysm sac contains a direct communication with the artery, which is characteristically turbulent in flow. They can result from catheterization, surgery, trauma, or inflammation. Pseudoaneurysms necessitate treatment because they can be a source of emboli, become infected, and rupture.[1–3]

Symptoms of pseudoaneurysm formation include a painful mass that may be pulsatile and can limit ambulation. Mass effect can cause localized ischemia, which can lead to overlaying skin and soft tissue necrosis. Compressive effects on local nerves can lead to neuralgia. Venous stasis and edema caused by mass effect on the femoral vein can lead to deep vein thrombosis. Less common but more serious complications include rupture and hemorrhage.[1–4]

Of the complications of femoral artery catheterization, pseudoaneurysm formation is the most common, comprising 61%.[2] Pseudoaneurysms occur in 0.11% to 1.52% of arterial catheterizations.[4–6] The incidence in diagnostic-only studies is 0.1% to 1.1%.[2,4] The overall incidence of pseudoaneurysm formation increases with therapeutic catheter interventions, occurring in 3.5% to 5.5%.[2] This is likely caused by the increased manipulation, length of time, and increased size of the arterial defect required for therapeutic intervention. A low puncture site is also considered a risk factor for pseudoaneurysm formation.[2]

Ultrasound (US) is often the initial tool used for diagnosis (Fig. 1A). This modality is an inexpensive and readily available method to make a fast diagnosis. US is noninvasive and requires no renal-harming contrast material. It is useful in the differentiation of the various postcatheterization complications; pseudoaneurysm versus arteriovenous (AV) fistula or hematoma formation. Additional diagnostic modalities include CT angiography (Fig. 2A, B) and MR angiography.[1,3,7]

[a] Department of Radiology, University of Virginia Health System, Charlottesville, VA, USA; [b] Division of Vascular Interventional Radiology, Department of Radiology and Imaging Sciences, University of Virginia Health System, Charlottesville, VA, USA
* Corresponding author.
E-mail address: NH6Y@Virginia.edu

Ultrasound Clin 7 (2012) 299–307
doi:10.1016/j.cult.2012.03.009

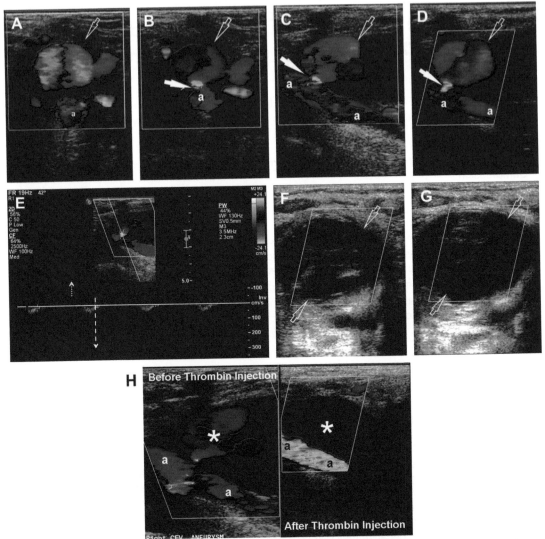

Fig. 1. (*A*) Doppler ultrasound on the right groin at the level of the common femoral artery (a) after a hepatic artery transplant angiogram. The patient is on steroids, antiplatelet therapy, and anticoagulants. The transducer is transverse to the common femoral artery (a). The pseudoaneurysm (PSA) (*open arrow*) is superficial to the common femoral artery (a) and displays the typical "ying-yang" sign. (*B*) A more cephalad Doppler US scan (transducer still transverse) at the level of the PSA neck (*solid arrow*). The PSA (*open arrow*) superficial to the common femoral artery (a). The PSA is still showing the classic "ying-yang" sign. (*C*) Doppler US on the right groin with the transducer longitudinal to the common femoral artery (a). The PSA (*open arrow*) is seen superficial to the common femoral artery (a). The *solid arrow* points to the base of the neck of the PSA. (*D*) Longitudinal image of the Doppler ultrasound on the right groin at the level of the common femoral artery (a) with the transducer longitudinal to the common femoral artery (a). The PSA (*open arrow*) is seen superficial to the common femoral artery (a). The *solid arrow* points to the base of the neck of the PSA. (*E*) Doppler US spectral waveform analysis focused on the PSA neck. The "yin-yang" is represented by the intermittent bidirectional arterial flow to-and-fro in the PSA neck. This is represented in the waveform analysis with flow above (*dotted arrow*) and below (*dashed arrow*) the 0 cm/s line. (*F*) Doppler US on the right groin over the PSA (between *open arrows*) after percutaneous needle thrombin injection into the PSA. There is no flow (color-coded flow) seen. (*G*) Another image of the Doppler US on the right groin over the PSA (between *open arrows*) after percutaneous needle thrombin injection into the PSA. There is no flow (color-coded flow) seen in the PSA. (*H*) Doppler US images of the right groin before (*left*) and after (*right*) percutaneous thrombin injection. The PSA (*asterisk*) has been completely obliterated after the thrombin injection (*right*). The common femoral artery (a) is preserved.

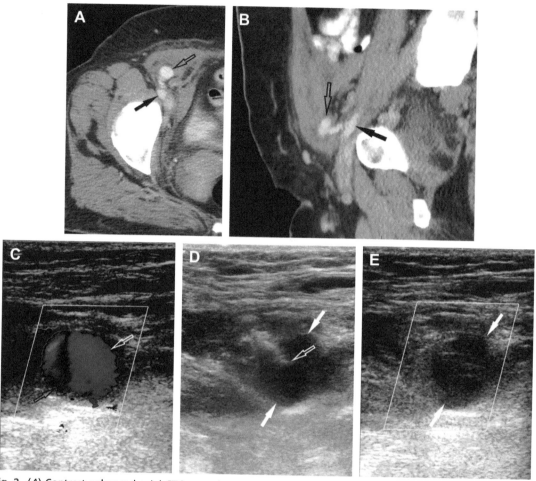

Fig. 2. (*A*) Contrast-enhanced axial CT image demonstrating a PSA (*open arrow*) off the common femoral artery (*solid arrow*). (*B*) Contrast-enhanced CT (saggital reformat) demonstrating the PSA (*open arrow*) off the common femoral artery (*solid arrow*). (*C*) Color Doppler US image demonstrating a PSA (between *open arrows*) with the classic "ying-yang" sign. (*D*) Gray-scale US image with the needle tip (*open arrow*) in the center of the PSA (between *solid arrows*). (*E*) Color Doppler US image demonstrating no flow within the PSA (between *solid arrows*).

Historically, pseudoaneurysms were treated with surgery. Newer methods include endoluminal approaches, US-guided compression, and percutaneous thrombin injection. Currently, the most commonly used techniques are direct percutaneous thrombin injection and US-guided compression.[7–9]

SONOGRAPHIC APPEARANCE OF PSEUDOANEURYSMS

US is the initial modality of choice for postcatheterization pseudoaneurysm diagnosis and treatment guidance. Gray-scale US images show a cystic or lobulated, hypoechoic region adjacent to a donor artery (see **Fig. 2**A–E). The cystic portion (pseudoaneurysm sac), is typically connected to the supplying artery by a relatively narrow communication (neck), demonstrating bidirectional

flow on color-flow Doppler US. Pseudoaneurysms can be described as simple (containing one lobe) or complex (more than one lobe). Color-flow Doppler US of the pseudoaneurym sac characteristically demonstrates turbulent, swirling flow often described as the "yin-yang sign." Differentiation of pseudoaneurysm from other postcatheterization groin masses, such as hematoma and iatrogenic AV fistula, is important because of differing management approaches for each diagnosis.[1,3,7,8]

PSEUDOANEURYSM COMPRESSION
Indications

Compression techniques have shown to be most successful in nonobese, nonanticoagulated patients with small pseudoaneurysms with a long neck. Ideally, pseudoaneurysms should be less than 2 weeks old. There should not be any overlaying skin breakdown. If possible, patients should be taken off anticoagulant therapy because of the decreased rate of treatment success. Large pseudoaneurysms have been associated with extended compression times and lower success rates.[10–12]

Contraindications

Contraindications to pseudoaneurysm compression include the following: pain intolerance, morbid obesity, anticoagulation therapy, large pseudoaneurysms, associated AV fistula component, overlying skin breakdown or infection, and unstable patients.

Technique

Fellmeth and coworkers[13] initially described US-guided compression of pseudoaneurysms in 1991. Several different methods of pseudoaneurysm compression are mentioned in the literature. These methods include blind compression without image guidance, real-time US-guided compression, and real-time guided US pseudoaneurysm neck compression. Additionally, the use of the vice-like FemoStop (St. Jude Medical, St. Paul, MN, USA) device has been described.[14]

The most commonly used method of compression is real-time US-guided pseudoaneurysm neck compression.[10–12,15] Before compression, US is used to evaluate the size, pseudoaneurysm neck location, amount of lobes, and flow characteristics. US is also needed to evaluate for any AV fistula component. The route of compression is also planned to apply maximal pressure on the pseudoaneurysm neck, while avoiding the pseudoaneurysm sac and femoral vessels. The distal arterial pulses are evaluated before the procedure. Certain patients may require moderate sedation to tolerate compression.

Pressure is applied by the US probe in a trajectory that compresses the pseudoaneurysm neck until flow has ceased. Care is taken to avoid compressing the adjacent femoral artery. Occasionally, the pseudoaneurysm neck cannot be clearly delineated. In these cases, direct US-guided compression of the pseudoaneurysm sac is preformed. Compression is applied in time intervals of 6 to 20 minutes.[6,8,16] Between compression intervals, the pseudoaneurysm is evaluated for internal flow using color-flow Doppler US. Compression is repeated until the pseudoaneurysm has been thrombosed. A maximum of three to four compression intervals are typically attempted before aborting. The limitations of the technique include patient pain intolerance and operator fatigue because of the extended manual compression that is often required.

After the pseudoaneurysm has been successfully thrombosed, the distal arterial pulses are evaluated and compared with the preprocedural evaluation. The patient is to remain on bed rest for the next 4 to 6 hours. Follow-up color-flow Doppler US is then completed within the next 24 hours.

Complications

The most common complications of pseudoaneurysm compression are related to the pain of the procedure itself. Additional complications include the likely cardiovascular responses to pain (hypotension, hypertension, atrial fibrillation, and chest angina). The use of moderate sedation can greatly reduce these complications. Rare complications include deep vein thrombosis, distal arterial embolization, and pseudoaneurysm rupture.[9,11,12,15]

Outcomes

Compression treatment of pseudoaneurysms was found to be effective in 80% of cases drawn from 47 studies.[4–6,9,14–60] The initial attempt effectiveness of compression therapy is 73%. A substantial amount of eventual successes required more than one attempt (13%). Typical reported total procedure times for compression therapy range from 37 to 75 minutes, with an average of 61 minutes. The rate of overall complications is 1.3%, with most (0.7%) being pain related.

DIRECT PERCUTANEOUS THROMBIN INJECTION
Indications

US-guided percutaneous thrombin injection has become the technique of choice for treatment of postcatheterization pseudoaneurysms at most institutions because of its high rate of success and relatively low complication rates.[1,3,5]

Contraindications

Contraindications to direct percutaneous thrombin injection include the following: associated AV fistula component, infected pseudoaneurysms, overlying skin breakdown, ruptured pseudoaneurysm, ipsilateral deep vein thrombosis, and allergy to thrombin.

Equipment

Equipment used in direct percutaneous thrombin injection includes US with a linear-array transducer (5–7.5 MHz); needle (20–22 gauge most commonly used); and thrombosing agent. The types of thrombosing agent available are bovine-derived thrombin and human-derived thrombin.

Technique

Initially, the distal arteries are evaluated by palpation, Doppler, or ankle-brachial index. Additionally, the overlying skin is evaluated for breakdown and infection. The pseudoaneurysm is then characterized by color-flow Doppler US. The size, number of lobes, flow dynamics, and pseudoaneurysm neck are evaluated. Assessment for associated AV components is also indicated. The needle approach is then decided based on the pseudoaneurysm shape, characteristics, and adjacent anatomy. Ideally, the needle tip is positioned in the pseudoaneurysm sac as far from the neck as accessible. Regarding multilobulated pseudoaneurysms (complex), there is persistent disagreement as to injecting the more proximal verses the distal lobe first. The concentration of thrombin used ranges from 100 to 1000 U/mL.[5,7,8]

The procedural site and US probe are prepared and draped in the standard fashion. Using gray-scale US, the needle tip is guided into the pseudoaneurysm sac (**Fig. 3**B, C). After the needle tip

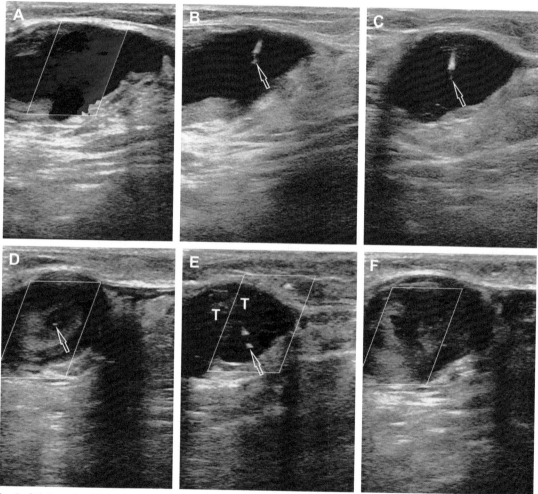

Fig. 3. (*A*) Doppler US of the groin showing an access PSA. (*B*) Gray-scale US of the same groin during percutaneous thrombin injection (just before the injection) showing the needle (*open arrow* at needle-tip) in the center of the PSA. (*C*) Gray-scale US of the same groin during percutaneous thrombin injection (just before the injection) showing the needle (*open arrow* at needle-tip) in the center of the PSA. (*D*) Doppler US during percutaneous thrombin injection showing the needle in the center of the PSA (*open arrow*) with new thrombus formation. The halo around the needle is from the continuous (minimal) thrombin injection making a "clearing" around the needle. (*E*) The needle tip (*open arrow* at needle tip) has been repositioned within PSA in one of the thrombus-free pockets for additional thrombin injection. The other quadrants of the PSA are thrombosed (T). (*F*) Doppler US showing complete obliteration of the PSA.

is in the ideal location, thrombin is injected slowly while under direct visualization using color-flow Doppler. While injecting, hyperechoic thrombus is formed within the pseudoaneurysm sac. The rate needs to be slow enough to avoid excessive thrombin reflux into the donor artery, but fast enough to avoid encasement of the needle tip by thrombus (see **Fig. 3**D). Needle tip encasement by thrombus can impede further injection. When this happens, careful movement of the needle tip can free this thrombus into the pseudoaneurysm sac (see **Fig. 3**E). Pseudoaneurysm thrombosis usually occurs in a matter of seconds after thrombin is injected (see **Fig. 3**F). Infrequently, there are several areas of incomplete thrombosis within the sac. These areas are typically allowed to thrombose on their own, as long as they do not contain significant flow. High-flow pockets within a thrombosed pseudoaneurysm may necessitate further direct thrombin injection.

Postprocedural care involves placing a pressure dressing over the site. Evaluation of the downstream arteries is then compared with the preprocedural examination for assessment of distal embolization. Most centers recommend postprocedural bed rest, although the duration varies between 1 and 24 hours. Follow-up US study is usually completed within 24 hours to evaluate if further intervention is needed.

Complications

Distal arterial embolization is the most frequently occurring and worrisome adverse effect. Nearly one-third of these embolic events require further treatment.[16] This complication is likely caused by reflux of thrombin into the femoral artery. Although the absolute prevention of thrombin reflux into the femoral artery is difficult to avoid, minimal leakage of thrombin is likely tolerated because of inactivation by circulating antithrombin III and dilution within the systemic bloodstream.[61] Using a less concentrated thrombin, 100 instead of 1000 U/mL, could potentially reduce the risk of distal arterial embolic events.[62] Additional possible complications include pain, pseudoaneurysm rupture, and allergic reaction.[5,7,8] The risk of an allergic reaction most likely increases with previous exposure to bovine thrombin. Allergic reactions can be avoided by using human-derived thrombin.[1]

OUTCOMES

Direct percutaneous thrombin injection treatment of pseudoaneurysms was considered a success in 97% of cases drawn from 36 studies containing 1722 pseudoaneurysms.[5,14,16,26,28,29,31,33–35,42,51–56,63–82] The initial attempt success was found to be 89%.

The overall average procedure time was found to be 21 minutes. The most common complication of direct thrombin injection therapy is distal arterial embolization, which occurs in 1% of cases. About 29% of the distal arterial embolization events eventually required dedicated treatment.

As demonstrated, direct thrombin injection has several advantages over compression therapy including decreased total procedure time (21 vs 61 minutes); higher overall success (97% vs 80%); and higher first attempt success (89% vs 73%). Other advantages of thrombin injection over compression therapy include higher patient tolerance, fewer patients ruled ineligible because of contraindications, and its ability to be successful when anticoagulation cannot be discontinued.

REFERENCES

1. Hanson JM, Atri M, Power N. Ultrasound-guided thrombin infection of iatrogenic groin pseudoaneurysm: Doppler features and technical tips. Br J Radiol 2008;81:154–63.
2. Kronzon I. Diagnosis and treatment of iatrogenic femoral artery pseudoaneurysm: a review. J Am Soc Echocardiogr 1997;10(3):236–45.
3. Saad NE, Saad WE, Davies MG, et al. Pseudoaneurysms and the role of minimally invasive techniques in their management. Radiographics 2005;25(Suppl 1): S173–89.
4. Atles M, Sahin S, Konuralp C, et al. Evaluation of risk factors associated with femoral pseudoaneurysms after cardiac catheterization. J Vasc Surg 2006;43: 520–4.
5. Olsen DM, Rodriguez JA, Vranic M, et al. A prospective study of ultrasound scan-guided thrombin injection of femoral pseudoaneurysm: a trend toward minimal medication. J Vasc Surg 2002;36:779–82.
6. Lange P, Houe T, Helgstrand UJ. The efficacy of ultrasound-guided compression of iatrogenic femoral pseudoaneurysms. Eur J Vasc Endovasc Surg 2001;21:248–50.
7. Morgan R, Belli A. Current treatment methods for postcatheterization pseudoaneurysms. J Vasc Interv Radiol 2003;14(6):697–710.
8. Middleton WD, Dasyam A, Teefey SA. Diagnosis and treatment of iatrogenic femoral artery pseudoaneurysms. Ultrasound Q 2005;21:3–17.
9. Paschalidis M, Thiess W, Kolling K, et al. Randomized comparison of manual compression repair versus ultrasound guided compression repair of postcatheterization femoral pseudoaneurysms. Heart 2004;92:251–2.
10. Chatterjee T, Do DD, Kaufmann U, et al. Ultrasound guided compression repair for treatment of femoral

artery pseudoaneurysm: acute and follow-up results. Cathet Cardiovasc Diagn 1996;38:335–40.

11. Coley BD, Roberts AC, Fellmeth BD, et al. Postangiographic femoral artery pseudoaneurysms: further experience with US-guided compression repair. Radiology 1995;194:307–11.

12. Cox GS, Young JR, Gray BR, et al. Ultrasound-guided compression repair of postcatheterization pseudoaneurysms: results of treatment in one hundred cases. J Vasc Surg 1994;19:683–6.

13. Fellmeth BD, Roberts AC, Bookstein JJ, et al. Postangiographic femoral artery injuries: nonsurgical repair with US-guided compression. Radiology 1991;178:671–5.

14. Chatterjee T, Do DD, Mahler F, et al. A prospective, randomized evaluation of nonsurgical closure of femoral pseudoaneurysm by compression device with or without ultrasound guidance. Catheter Cardiovasc Interv 1999;47:304–9.

15. Eisenberg L, Paulson EK, Kliewer MA, et al. Sonographically guided compression repair of pseudoaneurysms: further experience from a single institution. AJR Am J Roentgenol 1999;173(6): 1567–73.

16. Saad WE, Waldman DL. Management of postcatheterization pseudoaneurysms. In: Mauro MA, Murphy K, Thomson K, et al, editors. Image-guided interventions. Philadelphia (PA): Saunders/Elsevier; 2008. p. 525–36.

17. Chua TP, Howling SJ, Wright C, et al. Ultrasound-guided compression of femoral pseudoaneurysm: an audit of practice. Int J Cardiol 1998;63:245–50.

18. Perkins JM, Gordon AC, Magee TR, et al. Duplex-guided compression of femoral artery false aneurysms reduces the need for surgery. Ann R Coll Surg Engl 1996;78:473–5.

19. Lewis DR, Davies AH, Irvine CD, et al. Compression ultrasonography for false femoral artery aneurysm: hypocoagulability is a cause of failure. Eur J Vasc Endovasc Surg 1998;16:427–8.

20. Feld R, Patton GM, Carabasi RA, et al. Treatment of iatrogenic femoral artery injuries with ultrasound-guided compression. J Vasc Surg 1992;16:832–40.

21. Paulson EK, Kliewer MA, Hertzberg BS, et al. Ultrasonographically guided manual compression of femoral artery injuries. J Ultrasound Med 1995;14: 653–9.

22. Naimi A, Didier D, Grossholz M, et al. Treatment of post-coronarography femoral false aneurysm by compression, guided by Doppler echography. J Radiol 1996;77:247–52.

23. Veraldi GF, Furlan F, Benussi P, et al. Echo-guided compression in the treatment of femoral pseudoaneurysms secondary to cardiological interventional procedures. Chir Ital 1999;51:283–8.

24. Langella RL, Schneider JR, Golan JF. Color duplex-guided compression therapy for postcatheterization

pseudoaneurysms in a community hospital. Ann Vasc Surg 1996;10:27–35.

25. Pinto F, Lencioni R, Stringari R, et al. [Doppler color US in the diagnosis and treatment of iatrogenic pseudoaneurysms]. Radiol Med (Torino) 1997;94: 198–201 [in Italian].

26. Khoury M, Rebecca A, Greene K, et al. Duplex scanning-guided thrombin injection for the treatment of iatrogenic pseudoaneurysms. J Vasc Surg 2002; 35:517–21.

27. Ururluoglu A, Katzenschlager R, Ahmadi R, et al. Ultrasound guided compression therapy in 134 patients with iatrogenic pseudo-aneurysms: advantage of routine duplex ultrasound control of the puncture site following transfemoral catheterization. Vasa 1997;26:110–6.

28. Lonn L, Olmarker A, Gerterud K, et al. Treatment of femoral pseudoaneurysms: percutaneous US-guided thrombin injection verses US-guided compression. Acta Radiol 2002;43:396–400.

29. Pezzullo JA, Dupuy DE, Cronan JJ. Percutaneous injection of thrombin for the treatment of pseudoaneurysms after catheterization: an alternative to sonographically guided compression. AJR Am J Roentgenol 2000;175(4):1035–40.

30. Steinkamp HJ, Werk M, Felix R. Treatment of postinterventional pseudoaneurysms by ultrasound-guided compression. Invest Radiol 2000;35:186–92.

31. Lonn L, Olmarker A, Gerterud K, et al. Prospective randomized study comparing ultrasound-guided thrombin injection to compression in the treatment of femoral pseudoaneurysms. J Endovasc Ther 2004;11:570–6.

32. Chatterjee T, Do DD, Maher F, et al. Pseudoaneurysm of femoral artery after catheterization: treatment by a mechanical compression device guided by colour Doppler ultrasound. Heart 1998; 79:502–4.

33. McNeil NL, Clark TW. Sonographically guided percutaneous thrombin injection versus sonographically guided compression for femoral artery pseudoaneurysms. AJR Am J Roentgenol 2001;176: 459–62.

34. Weinmann EE, Chayen D, Kobzantzen ZV, et al. Treatment of postcatheterization false aneurysms: ultrasound-guided compression vs. ultrasound-guided thrombin injection. Eur J Vasc Endovasc Surg 2002;23:68–72.

35. Paulson EK, Sheafor DH, Kliewer MA, et al. Treatment of iatrogenic femoral arterial pseudoaneurysms: comparison of US-guided thrombin injection with compression repair. Radiology 2000;215:403–8.

36. Knight CG, Healy DA, Thomas RL. Femoral artery pseudoaneurysms: risk factors, prevalence, and treatment options. Ann Vasc Surg 2003;17:503–8.

37. Theiss W, Schreiber K, Schomig A. Manual compression repair of post-catheterization femoral

pseudoaneurysms: an alternative to ultrasound guided compression repair? Vasa 2002;31:95–9.

38. Murphy PB, Bajwa TK, Kubota J, et al. Peripheral artery pseudoaneurysm: treatment by trancutaneous compression guided by ultrasound. Echocardiography 1996;13:483–8.

39. Kubale R, Roman S, Abd-al-Maabud M, et al. [Pseudoaneurysms of the femoral artery: noninvaisive diagnosis and compression therapy]. Bildgebung 1993;60:135–9 [in German].

40. Elliott JM, Kelly IM. Ultrasound guided compression of femoral artery pseudoaneurysms: modified digital technique shortens repair time. Clin Radiol 1999;54:683–6.

41. Sillesen HH, Neilsen TG, Vogt KC. [Pseudoaneurysm of the femoral artery treated with color Doppler ultrasonography guided compression]. Ugeskr Laeger 1995;157:5101–3 [in Danish].

42. Gorge G, Kunz T, Kirstein M. A prospective study on ultrasound-guided compression therapy of thrombin injection for treatment of iatrogenic false aneuryms in patients receiving full-dose anti-platelet therapy. Z Kardiol 2003;92:564–70.

43. Engelhorn CA, Picheth FS, Castro-Junior N, et al. Treatment of femoral false aneurysms following cardiac catheterization with compression and color Doppler echocardiography monitoring. Arq Bras Cardiol 1997;68:429–31.

44. Feng YL, Truitt RE, Coggins TR, et al. Nonsurgical repair of femoral artery pseudoaneurysm with color flow guided ultrasound transducer compression. Echocardiography 1996;13:297–302.

45. Davies AH, Hayward JK, Irvine CD, et al. Short note: treatment of iatrogenic false aneurysm by compression ultrasonography. Br J Surg 1995;82:1230–1.

46. DiPrete DA, Cronan JJ. Compression ultrasonography: treatment for acute femoral artery pseudoaneurysm in selected cases. J Ultrasound Med 1992;11:489–92.

47. Seitz C, Kaddatz J, Kester M, et al. [Color Doppler-guided compression of pseudoaneurysms after arterial puncture: early and late results]. Dtsch Med Wochenschr 1995;120:205–8 [in German].

48. Hajarizadeh H, Larosa CR, Cardullo P, et al. Ultrasound-guided compression of iatrogenic femoral pseudoaneurysm failure, recurrence, and long-term results. J Vasc Surg 1995;22:425–30.

49. Oelerich M, Lentschig MG, Vestring T, et al. [The color Doppler-guided compression therapy of pseudoaneurysms: the author's own experiences and review of the literature]. Rofo 1996;165:484–90 [in German].

50. Moote DJ, Hilborn MD, Harris KA, et al. Postarteriographic femoral pseudoaneurysms: treatment with ultrasound-guided compression. Ann Vasc Surg 1994;8:325–31.

51. Ramsey DW, Marshall M. Treatment of iatrogenic femoral artery false aneurysms with ultrasound-guided thrombin injection. Australas Radiol 2002;46:264–6.

52. Demharter J, Leissner G, Huf V, et al. [Treatment of iatrogenic femoral pseudoaneurysms with thrombin injection: results in 54 patients]. Rofo 2005;177:550–4 [in German].

53. Maleux G, Hendrickx S, Vaninbroukx J, et al. Percutaneous injection of human thrombin to treat iatrogenic femoral pseudoaneurysms: short and midterm ultrasound followup. Eur Radiol 2003;13:209–12.

54. Loose HW, Haslam PJ. The management of peripheral arterial aneurysms using percutaneous injection of fibrin adhesive. Br J Radiol 1998;71:1255–9.

55. Matson MB, Morgan RA, Beli AM. Percutaneous treatment of pseudoaneurysms using fibrin adhesive. Br J Radiol 2001;74:690–4.

56. Owen RJ, Haslam PJ, Elliott ST, et al. Percutaneous ablation of peripheral pseudoaneurysms using thrombin: a simple and effective solution. Cardiovasc Intervent Radiol 2000;23:441–6.

57. Tarro-Genta F, Bevilacqua R, Bosimini E. Ultrasound-guided compression repair of femoral pseudoaneurysms complicating cardiac catheterization. Ital Heart J 2004;5:132–5.

58. Hood DB, Mattos MA, Douglas MG, et al. Determinants of success of color-flow duplex-guided compression repair of femeral pseudoaneurysms. Surgery 1996;120:588–90.

59. Szendro G, Klimov A, Lennox A, et al. [Femoral artery pseudo-aneurysms: change in treatment, report of 7-years]. Harefuah 2000;139:187–90 [in Hebrew].

60. Demirbas O, Guven A, Batyrallev T. Management of 28 consecutive iatrogenic femoral pseudoaneurysms with ultrasound guided compression. Heart Vessels 2005;20(3):91–4.

61. Grewe PH, Mugge A, Germig A, et al. Occlusion of pseudoaneurysms using human or bovine thrombin using contrast-enhanced ultrasound guidance. Am J Cardiol 2004;93:1540–2.

62. Sadiq S, Ibrahim W. Thromboembolism complicating thrombin injection of femoral artery pseudoaneurysm: management with intraarterial thrombolysis. J Vasc Interv Radiol 2001;12(5):633–6.

63. Vazquez V, Reus M, Pinero A, et al. Human thrombin for treatment of pseudoaneurysms: comparison of bovine and human thrombin sonogram-guided injection. AJR Am J Roentgenol 2005;184:1665–71.

64. Gale SS, Scissons RP, Jones L, et al. Remoral pseudoaneurysm thromboinjection. Am J Surg 2001;181:379–83.

65. Vermeulen EG, Umans U, Rijbroek A, et al. Percutaneous duplex-guided thrombin injection for treatment of iatrogenic femoral artery pseudoaneurysms. Eur J Vasc Endovasc Surg 2000;20:302–4.

66. Lennox AF, Delis KT, Szendro G, et al. Duplex-guided thrombin injection for iatrogenic femoral artery pseudoaneurysm is effective even in anticoagulated patients. Br J Surg 2000;87:796–801.

67. Quarmby JW, Engelke C, Chitolie A, et al. Autologous thrombin for treatment of pseudoaneurysms. Lancet 2002;359:946–7.

68. Hughes MJ, McCall JM, Nott DM, et al. Treatment of iatrogenic femoral artery pseudoaneurysms using ultrasound-guided injection of thrombin. Clin Radiol 2000;55:749–51.

69. Paulson EK, Nelson RC, Mayes CE, et al. Sonographically guided thrombin injection of iatrogenic femoral pseudoaneurysms: further experience at a single institution. AJR Am J Roentgenol 2001;177:309–16.

70. Sackett WR, Taylor SM, Coffey CB, et al. Ultrasound-guided thrombin injection of iatrogenic femoral pseudoaneurysms: a prospective analysis. Am Surg 2000;66:937–42.

71. Corso R, Rampoldi A, Riolo F, et al. Occlusion of postcatheterization femoral pseudoaneurysms with percutaneous thrombin injection under ultrasound guidance. Radiol Med (Torino) 2004;108:385–93.

72. Sheiman RG, Brophy DP. Treatment of iatrogenic femoral pseudoaneurysms with percutaneous thrombin injection: experience in 54 patients. Radiology 2001;219:123–7.

73. Sheiman RG, Mastromatteo M. Iatrogenic femoral pseudoaneurysms that are unresponsive to percutaneous thrombin injection: potential causes. AJR Am J Roentgenol 2003;181:1301–4.

74. La Perna L, Olin JW, Goines D, et al. Ultrasound-guided thrombin injection for the treatment of postcatheterization pseudoaneurysms. Circulation 2000;102:2391–5.

75. Stone P, Lohan JA, Copeland SE, et al. Iatrogenic pseudoaneurysms: comparison of treatment modalities, including duplex-guided thrombin injection. W V Med J 2003;99:230–2.

76. Taylor BS, Rhee RY, Muluk S, et al. Thrombin injection versus compression of femoral artery pseudoaneurysms. J Vasc Surg 1999;30:1052–9.

77. Gorge G, Kunz T. Thrombin injection for the treatment of false aneurysms after failed compression therapy in patients on full-dose antiplatelet and heparin therapy. Catheter Cardiovasc Interv 2003;58:505–9.

78. Edgerton JR, Moore DO, Nichols D, et al. Obliteration of femoral artery pseudoaneurysm by thrombin injection. Ann Thorac Surg 2002;74:S1413–5.

79. Grewe PH, Deneke T, Fadgyas T, et al. Minimally invasive percutaneous contrast-ultrasound guided thrombin occlusion of iatrogenic pseudoaneurysm. Z Kardiol 2001;90:737–44.

80. Mohler ERIII, Mitchell ME, Carpenter JP, et al. Therapeutic thrombin injection of pseudoaneurysms: a multicenter experience. Vasc Med 2001;6:241–4.

81. Elford J, Burrell C, Freeman S, et al. Human thrombin injection for the percutaneous treatment of iatrogenic pseudoaneurysms. Cardiovasc Intervent Radiol 2002;25:115–8.

82. Kang SS, Labropoulos N, Mansour A, et al. Percutaneous ultrasound guided thrombin injection: a new method for treating postcatheterization femoral pseudoaneurysms. J Vasc Surg 1998;27:1032–8.

Ultrasound-Guided Breast Interventions

Jennifer A. Harvey, MD*, Alecia W. Sizemore, MD

KEYWORDS

- Mammography • Fine-needle aspiration biopsy • Ultrasound-guided breast procedures
- Cyst aspiration

KEY POINTS

- Physicians performing ultrasound-guided breast procedures should be familiar with and fulfill qualifications outlined in the American College of Radiology Practice Guidelines for the Performance of Ultrasound-Guided Percutaneous Breast Interventional Procedures.
- Most breast lesions visible on ultrasonography are amenable to ultrasound-guided core biopsy, typically using an entry from the periphery of the breast that produces a path parallel to the chest wall.
- Fine-needle aspiration biopsy and cyst aspiration techniques use a short approach with the needle advancing toward the lesion at an angle of 30° to 45°.
- Postprocedure mammogram following placement of a radiopaque biopsy marker can confirm concordance between the sonographic and mammographic findings.
- Postprocedure patient follow-up includes performance and documentation of any delayed complications and treatment administered, radiologic-histologic correlation, and communication of biopsy results and recommendations to the patient and/or referring physician.

CLASSIFICATION

Ultrasound-guided breast interventions may be diagnostic, therapeutic, or both. Interventions include, but are not limited to:

- Percutaneous biopsy
  - Breast lesions
  - Axillary adenopathy
- Preoperative (wire) localization
- Cyst aspiration
- Abscess drainage.

The primary content of this article focuses on percutaneous ultrasound-guided breast biopsy using freehand guidance. Many of the concepts used for ultrasound-guided biopsy can be transferred to other ultrasound-guided interventions.

Ultrasound-guided needle biopsies can be classified as:

- Core-needle biopsy (CNB, automated throw needle)
  - Sensitivity of 97% to 99%
  - Can provide tissue sufficient for receptor status analysis
- Directional vacuum-assisted biopsy (DVAB, mammotomy)
- Fine-needle aspiration biopsy (FNAB):
  - Sensitivity and specificity of 85% to 88% and 56% to 90%, respectively, for non-palpable breast lesions
  - Can be useful in evaluating
    - Cystic lesions
    - Additional lesions or abnormal lymph nodes in the setting of a known primary breast cancer.

Division Head - Breast Imaging, University of Virginia Health System, Charlottesville, VA, USA
* Corresponding author.
E-mail address: jah7w@virginia.edu

Ultrasound Clin 7 (2012) 309–323
doi:10.1016/j.cult.2012.03.001
1556-858X/12/$ – see front matter © 2012 Published by Elsevier Inc.

GENERAL PRINCIPLES

Percutaneous image-guided biopsy has largely replaced diagnostic surgical biopsy in the evaluation of breast lesions in many practices. Compared with diagnostic surgical biopsy, percutaneous image-guided breast biopsy is:

- Less invasive, with reduced morbidity, better cosmetic results, and less scarring detectable on future breast imaging
- More efficient and less expensive than diagnostic surgical biopsy, with shorter recovery time
- Equivalent in accuracy to open surgical biopsy.

Once a malignancy has been diagnosed by percutaneous image-guided biopsy:

- The patient and surgeon are able to discuss therapeutic options in advance of a surgery.
- The extent of disease can be evaluated by ultrasonography or magnetic resonance (MR) imaging.
- Image-guided biopsy documenting multifocal or multicentric disease may alter surgical management.
- Percutaneous biopsy of nonpalpable malignancy results in a single therapeutic surgical operation in 81% of women.
- Receptor status as determined by CNB or DVAB samples can also guide neoadjuvant chemotherapy, if needed.

Advantages of ultrasound guidance for percutaneous breast biopsy over stereotactic guidance include:

- Lack of ionizing radiation, which is particularly important for pregnant women with a breast mass
- Real-time visualization of the needle during biopsy improves confidence that a small lesion has been accurately sampled
- Supine positioning is often more comfortable than prone, lateral decubitus, or sitting positions used for stereotactic procedures
- Stereotactic biopsy can be limited by a compressed breast thickness of at least 2.5 cm, whereas small breast thickness rarely affects the ability to perform ultrasound-guided breast biopsy
- In experienced hands, ultrasound-guided breast biopsies are often more efficient than stereotactic biopsy.

TRAINING

The American College of Radiology (ACR) Practice Guidelines for the Performance of Ultrasound-Guided Percutaneous Breast Interventional Procedures define qualifications and responsibilities for radiologists who perform these procedures (**Boxes 1 and 2**). Initial qualifications can be completed during residency or fellowship training programs.

INDICATIONS

Indications for ultrasound-guided breast interventions include:

- **Simple and complicated cysts,** when:
  - Symptomatic
  - Complicated cyst is suspected, but mass may be solid and is new or enlarging
  - Abscess is suspected, and therapeutic drainage is clinically indicated.
- **Complex and solid masses,** when:
  - Mass is assessed as suspicious (Breast Imaging Reporting and Data System [BI-RADS] assessment category 4) or highly suggestive of malignancy (BI-RADS 5)
  - Presence of more than 1 suspicious mass, to facilitate treatment planning.

Box 1
Principles from the ACR Practice Guideline for the Performance of Ultrasound-Guided Percutaneous Breast Interventional Procedures

Initial training:

Fulfill qualifications specified in the ACR Practice Guidelines for Performance of a Breast Ultrasound Examination (see **Box 2**)

Be capable of correlating results of mammography, other procedures, and the biopsy pathology with the sonographic findings, or review these results with a qualified physician

Obtain a minimum of 8 hours of continuing medical education (CME) in breast ultrasound-guided biopsy techniques

Perform at least 12 ultrasound-guided biopsy procedures under direct supervision

Thereafter, the ACR recommends that radiologists:

Perform at least 24 ultrasound-guided procedures every 2 years to maintain skills

Obtain at minimum of 3 hours of CME in ultrasound-guided breast biopsy every 3 years

○ Masses visualized on targeted ultrasound examination that correlate with a suspicious area of enhancement on breast MR imaging (BI-RADS 4 or 5)
○ Lesions with BI-RADS assessment category 3: Probably benign, are typically *not* biopsied under image guidance unless:

■ Accompanied by undue patient anxiety
■ Questionable reliability of the patient for return visit; for example, a homeless woman with limited health care resources
■ In the setting of a palpable finding, diagnostic ultrasound-guided biopsy can be an alternative to excision.

• **Repeat biopsy:**
○ Repeat percutaneous core or vacuum-assisted needle biopsy is an alternative to surgical biopsy in cases where an initial core biopsy is nondiagnostic or yields results that are discordant with the imaging findings; or if an initial FNAB results in atypical, suspicious, or nondiagnostic cytology.

• **Preoperative localization:**
○ When visible sonographically, ultrasound-guided localization can be performed for a lesion or marking device placed during previous biopsy.

• **Abnormal axillary lymph nodes** in cases of known or suspected malignancy:
○ Can be performed at the time of initial imaging-guided core biopsy of the suspicious breast mass, or at a later time
○ May reduce the number of women undergoing sentinel lymph node biopsy:
■ In the setting of locally advanced or metastatic breast cancer, biopsy of axillary lymph nodes showing metastatic breast cancer may document extent of disease before neoadjuvant chemotherapy
■ If FNA or core biopsy of an axillary lymph node in a woman with diagnosed or suspected breast cancer shows metastatic breast cancer before surgery, she may undergo axillary dissection at the first surgical procedure. The role of axillary lymph node sampling is evolving. Ultrasound-guided biopsy may not be indicated even when an axillary lymph node appears abnormal.

• **Axillary adenopathy** of unknown cause:
○ Can undergo diagnostic percutaneous ultrasound-guided biopsy:
■ In the setting of a known malignancy, FNA of an abnormal lymph node is typically adequate
■ When there is no known malignancy, CNB may be needed to exclude lymphoma.

• **Microcalcifications:**
Should typically undergo sampling using stereotactic guidance; however, if visible on ultrasonography, microcalcifications can undergo

ultrasound-guided biopsy when stereotactic guidance is not feasible (ie, limitations of breast size or patient positioning) (**Fig. 1**).

CONTRAINDICATIONS

Contraindications to ultrasound-guided breast biopsy include:

- Inability to visualize the biopsy target by ultrasonography
- Uncertainty that the ultrasonography finding correlates to suspicious finding on screening modality (ie, mammogram or MR imaging)
- Uncooperative patient during the procedure
  - If necessary, mild sedation using fast-acting oral agents can be helpful
- Uncorrectable bleeding diathesis
  - In these cases, FNAB or surgical biopsy may be preferred alternatives
- Breast implants
  - Can increase complexity of approach, but is not necessarily a contraindication to ultrasound-guided biopsy.

Not all lesions will be amenable to percutaneous image-guided biopsy. The literature reports the most commonly cited reasons for lesions not diagnosed by percutaneous biopsy:

- Difficulty visualizing lesion for image-guided biopsy
- Patient preference
- Lesion superficial or very small.

Mammography findings such as architecture distortion and calcifications, and MR imaging findings such as foci and non–mass enhancement may be difficult to identify on ultrasonography. Compared with ultrasonography, if a lesion is more confidently visualized on mammography or MR imaging, respectively, then image-guided biopsy by that modality is likely the better choice to improve confidence that the correct area was sampled (**Fig. 2**).

PREPROCEDURAL EVALUATION

- A complete diagnostic imaging workup should be performed and assessed by

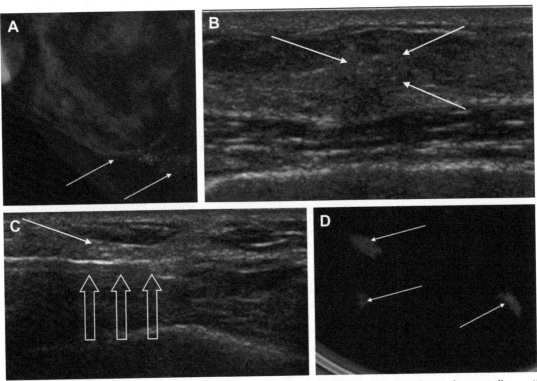

Fig. 1. A 66-year-old woman with suspicious microcalcifications on mammography who underwent diagnostic ultrasound-guided core-needle biopsy. Stereotactic-guided biopsy could not be performed because of small compressed breast thickness. (*A*) Mediolateral magnification view of the right breast shows fine pleomorphic calcifications in a linear distribution (*arrows*). (*B*) The calcifications were visualized on ultrasonography (*arrows*). (*C*) Ultrasound-guided vacuum-assisted biopsy (DVAB) was performed by placing the needle (*open arrows*) posterior to the calcifications (*white arrow*). (*D*) Specimen radiograph contains numerous calcifications (*arrows*). Histology revealed ductal carcinoma in situ.

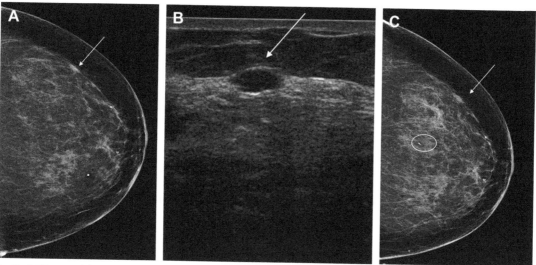

Fig. 2. A 61-year-old woman with abnormal left mammogram. (*A*) Left craniocaudal (CC) view shows a 6-mm oval mass with ill-defined margins (*arrow*). (*B*) Ultrasonography shows a corresponding 5-mm lobular hypoechoic solid mass in the left breast at 5 o'clock (*arrow*). (*C*) Postprocedure CC view shows that the clip (*circle*) is located approximately 3 cm from the lesion seen on mammogram (*arrow*). Core biopsy was therefore repeated using stereotactic guidance. Histology from both biopsies demonstrated intraductal papilloma.

a physician qualified to interpret the examination before scheduling a procedure, which:

- ○ Satisfies ACR Practice Guideline recommendations.
- ○ Improves efficiency of the procedure schedule, as no additional diagnostic imaging need be obtained that would result in delay or canceling of the procedure.
- Communication regarding need for biopsy, procedural information, and an appointment can be given to the patient by the radiologist and an on-site nurse or technologist at the time of diagnostic imaging.
- A list of the patient's medications should be reviewed before scheduling the biopsy appointment. Management of anticoagulant medication is coordinated with the prescribing physician. Although not mandated, the authors request patients discontinue their use of aspirin and nonsteroidal anti-inflammatory medications for 5 days before the procedure, if possible.
- On the day of the procedure:
  - ○ Informed consent can be obtained by the radiologist or a nurse.
  - ○ When consent is obtained, patients are queried regarding known vascular disease or diabetes to avoid the use of epinephrine in the local anesthesia to reduce the risk of skin injury.
  - ○ The possibility of surgery is discussed with the patient should the CNB pathology

show a benign high-risk lesion (ie, atypical ductal hyperplasia or radial scar). If a high-risk lesion is indeed detected by CNB, this practice forewarns the patient that surgery is a possible recommendation even if the CNB did not show cancer.

- After the procedure, the physician performing the procedure is responsible for:
  - ○ Documenting the procedure and any complications with treatment administered
  - ○ Obtaining the pathology results to determine adequacy of the biopsy and concordance or discordance of the biopsy results with respect to imaging findings
  - ○ Communicating biopsy results and recommendations to the referring physician and/or to the patient, as appropriate

EQUIPMENT
High-Frequency Linear Array Transducers

- A 10-MHz or higher linear transducer is highly recommended.
- Focal zones should be adjustable rather than fixed in position.

Needle Selection (Core Versus Vacuum)

Either automated throw needle (CNB) or DVAB devices can be used for ultrasound-guided breast biopsy.

Core-Needle Biopsy

- 14-gauge needles are most commonly used, but needle sizes range from 12-gauge to 18-gauge.
- Higher diagnostic yields have been demonstrated for 14-gauge needles compared with 16- or 18-gauge needles.

Vacuum-Assisted Biopsy (DVAB, Mammotomy)

- Needle sizes range from 8-gauge to 14-gauge.
- DVAB devices may collect single samples that must be retrieved after each needle pass (similar to CNB devices) or may collect multiple samples with a single needle insertion.
- DVAB is advantageous for selective cases:
  - Calcifications are more easily sampled using DVAB (see **Fig. 1**). The use of a core needle introduces air that quickly obscures the calcifications on ultrasonography.
  - A small or cystic lesion that may be difficult to visualize after the first 1 or 2 samples. In these cases, the needle can be placed deep (posterior) to the lesion and kept stationary during the biopsy. The lesion can be observed for resolution during real-time sampling.
- Bleeding complications may be slightly higher with DVAB devices than with CNB devices.

Fine-Needle Aspiration Biopsy

- 22-gauge spinal needles are typically used.
- FNAB has overall sensitivity considerably lower than CNB, and lower sensitivity for invasive lobular carcinoma compared with invasive ductal carcinoma.
- CNB should be performed instead of FNAB for most breast lesions.
- FNAB can be useful in:
  - Evaluation of cystic lesions of the breast. A complicated or possible hemorrhagic cyst may initially undergo aspiration. If a residual solid component remains, CNB can then be performed.
  - Evaluation of suspicious axillary lymph nodes (**Fig. 3**). FNAB of a suspicious node can circumvent the need for sentinel node biopsy in the setting of known breast cancer.
  - In the setting of a known or suspected primary breast cancer, additional lesions suspicious for invasive carcinoma can undergo FNAB or CNB to document the extent of disease.

ROOM SETUP

Before the start of the procedure, diagnostic breast imaging studies including mammograms, ultrasonograms, and MR images should be reviewed.

- Adjustable examination tables can be useful.
  - Variable height settings accommodate differing radiologist statures.
  - A table that pivots enables the radiologist to use dominant hand to manipulate the biopsy device, if desired. The examination table can be reversed to place the patient's head at the opposite end. This action alters the access path without losing the ability to view the ultrasound screen.

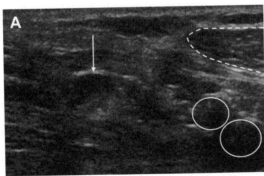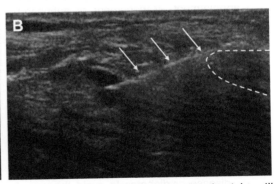

Fig. 3. Ultrasound-guided fine-needle aspiration technique. (*A*) Suspicious lymph node (*arrow*) in the right axilla of a 51-year-old woman with recent diagnosis of right invasive breast cancer. Note that the lymph node lies adjacent to the pectoralis muscle (*dashed line*) and axillary vessels (*circles*). (*B*) A steep needle angle (*arrows*) is used to avoid the pectoralis muscle (*dashed line*). The tip of the needle is within the cortex of the lymph node. Cytology showed reactive lymph node. The patient underwent sentinel node biopsy at time of surgery.

- Room lights should be dim enough to visualize the lesion well on the ultrasound screen. A second light source may be beneficial to adequately visualize skin marking(s) and dermatotomy.

PATIENT POSITIONING, PROCEDURE PREPARATION, AND DRAPING

- The patient lies supine on the examination table.
  - The ipsilateral arm is placed above the head.
  - The breast is scanned to localize the lesion of interest. Image settings should be optimized: depth adjusted, focal zones set at the area of interest, and gain set appropriately.
  - If the lesion is lateral and/or the breast large, wedge supports can be used to create an oblique position thereby enabling a more strategic transducer position with respect to the lesion.
- In planning the biopsy approach, the natural curvature of the breast can be used to advantage.
  - Visualization of the needle is optimal when perpendicular to the ultrasound beam, which occurs when the needle is parallel to the surface of the transducer.

- If the surface of the transducer is placed parallel to the chest wall, needle entry from the periphery of the breast yields a path that is both perpendicular to the ultrasound beam and parallel to the pectoralis muscle, reducing risk of chest wall injury (**Fig. 4**).
- Once the approach is decided, a "T" mark is drawn on the breast denoting the edge of the transducer and the anticipated needle entry site (**Fig. 5**A).
- The skin around the T mark and the location of the lesion is cleansed with an iodine solution. The use of a sterile eye-drape with an adhesive back (Steri-Drape; 3M, St. Paul, MN, USA) can be helpful in ensuring a clean field without the drape shifting in position during the procedure (see **Fig. 5**B).
- The transducer is likewise covered with a sterile cover (IsoSilk; Microtech, Columbus, MS) or cleansed with an antiseptic solution.

TECHNIQUE

- Before the procedure begins, the patient's identity, lesion laterality, procedure name/type, and patient's willingness to proceed should be verbally confirmed.
- Images should be labeled with the patient's name and at least one other identifier, as well as the name and location of the facility,

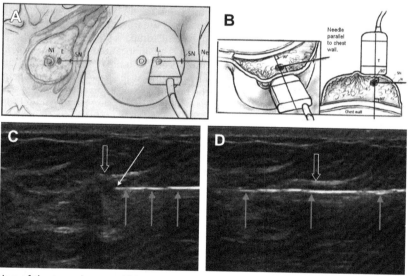

Fig. 4. Positioning of the transducer and biopsy needle. (*A*) The dermatotomy is made at the side of the breast in the same plane as the transducer. (*B*) Using this approach, the needle will be parallel to the chest wall and perpendicular to the ultrasound beam, which optimizes needle visualization. (*C*) Prefire ultrasound image, with the needle tip (*white arrow*) positioned at near edge of the lesion (*open arrow*). Note that the needle (*gray arrows*) is parallel to the surface of the transducer and chest wall. (*D*) Postfire ultrasound image, confirming that the needle (*gray arrows*) has traversed the lesion (*open arrow*).

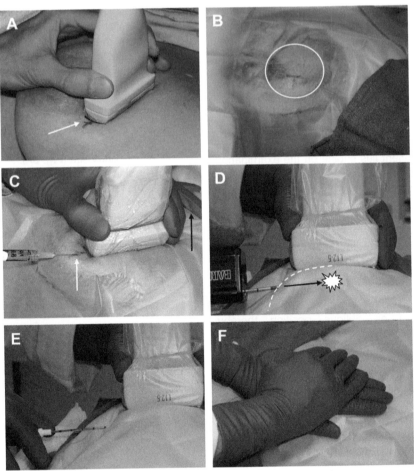

Fig. 5. Ultrasound-guided core needle biopsy method. (*A*) Typically, a lateral approach is easiest. Once the lesion is located and an approach is decided, a "T" is drawn on the breast (*arrow*) with the top of the T at the side of the transducer and the vertical portion of the T marking the plane of the transducer. The base of the T is made at the approximate depth of the lesion. (*B*) The skin is cleansed. A sterile drape is placed with the aperture (*circle*) over the area of the lesion to the bottom of the T. (*C*) The lesion is again localized using the T mark. Note that the index finger and thumb are located at the base of the transducer, while the remaining fingers anchor the transducer position (*black arrow*). Local anesthetic is injected by entering at the base of the T (*white arrow*). (*D*) After a dermatotomy is made, the biopsy needle is placed in the breast, also entering at the base of the T. Entry at the lateral curvature of the breast (*dashed line*) results in the needle (*black arrow*) being parallel to the face of the transducer as it approaches the lesion (*drawn white mass*). Further throw of the needle when fired to obtain a sample will not result in injury to the chest wall using this position. (*E*) A marker is placed after the samples are obtained using the same path as the biopsy needle. Note the positioning of the transducer has remained stable and unchanged during the entire procedure. (*F*) Following the procedure, manual pressure is placed over the entire needle path, which includes the dermatotomy and area of the lesion. (*Courtesy of* Dennis Sizemore.)

and the initials of the technologist and physician performing the procedure.

CORE-NEEDLE BIOPSY

- While establishing rapport with the patient, it may be beneficial to:
  - Demonstrate potentially startling noises to the patient, such as the sound of an automated throw needle device.
  - Consider use of the terms "biopsy device" and "sample" in place of "gun" and "fire," respectively, which may help to reduce patient anxiety.
- The transducer is held in one hand and the biopsy device in the other (see **Fig. 5**). Using the dominant hand for either function is a useful skill to develop.
- Align the long axis of the transducer with the lesion and the dermatotomy to define

the planned trajectory of the biopsy needle (see **Figs. 4** and **5D**).

- It is important to maintain constant visualization of the lesion from the time of local anesthesia injection until the biopsy marker is placed.
- Small or cystic lesions may be difficult to visualize after injection of local anesthesia or after the first sample is obtained (**Fig. 6**).
- The transducer must therefore maintain a steady, stable position.

- Hold the long axis of the transducer base between the thumb and index finger. Stabilize the position of the transducer by fanning out the fourth and fifth fingers along the breast (see **Fig. 5C**).
- Local anesthesia is established by injecting lidocaine (2%) in the skin, along the anticipated needle path and beyond the far side of the lesion. The needle path can go through solid lesions; however, it is advisable to avoid puncturing cystic lesions while anesthetizing.
  - The buffering of lidocaine, an acidic compound, may reduce pain associated with injection. Buffering can be accomplished by adding sodium bicarbonate (8.4%) in a volume ratio of 10:1 (5 mL lidocaine with 0.5 mL bicarbonate).
  - Lidocaine with epinephrine (1:100,000) can be used to reduce bleeding during the procedure.
    - An injection of lidocaine with epinephrine in the skin or a terminal capillary bed may result in focal necrosis.
    - Avoid using lidocaine with epinephrine in women who may have compromised vasculature, such as those with diabetes, known vascular disease, prior radiation therapy to the breast, or if the lesion is close to the skin.

- Form a dermatotomy with a single pass of an 11-blade incision scalpel.
- Insert the biopsy needle a short distance into the breast, just deep enough to identify the leading edge of the needle.
  - While maintaining transducer alignment along the path defined by the dermatotomy and the lesion, a tiny sweeping motion of the needle should bring the needle into the plane of the transducer resulting in visualization of the needle shaft (**Fig. 7**).
  - Minimizing downward pressure on the "thumb side" of the transducer may also aid in earlier visualization of the needle.
  - Once the needle is identified, make adjustments to the depth or angle before advancing the needle toward the lesion.

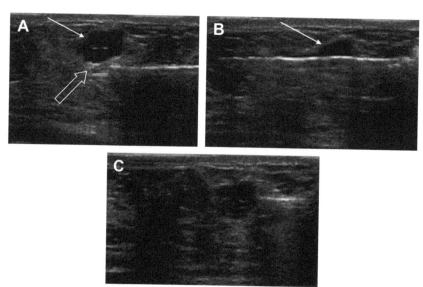

Fig. 6. A 41-year-old woman with a mass on baseline mammography (*not shown*). (*A*) A corresponding complex mass with predominantly cystic components is shown on ultrasonography (*arrow*). A biopsy marker was placed posterior to the complex mass before the biopsy (*open arrow*). (*B*) Postfire image after the first pass shows the needle traversing the lesion (*arrow*), in region of septations. (*C*) Prefire image for the second pass demonstrates partial resolution of the mass. Histology showed a cyst with acute inflammation.

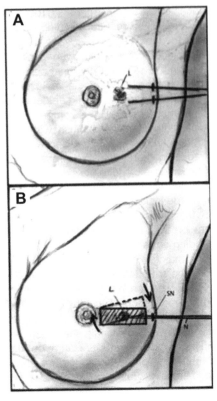

Sweeping motion to bring needle into plane of the transducer

(Keep transducer fixed)

Realign lesion and dermatotomy along long axis of transducer

SN = Dermatotomy (Skin Nick)
N = Needle
L = Lesion

Fig. 7. Visualizing the needle. (A) If the transducer is lined up with the lesion and dermatotomy, a small sweeping motion of the needle will bring the needle into the plane of the transducer. (B) If the needle is not visualized using this technique, the lesion is realigned with the dermatotomy by rotating the transducer. SN, dermatotomy (skin nick); N, needle; L, lesion.

- o Difficulty in identifying the needle during the procedure is usually due to lack of alignment of the needle and transducer. Look down at the relationship between the dermatotomy, needle, and transducer to facilitate this correction. Either the needle position can be adjusted or the transducer can be rotated to improve visualization of the needle (see **Fig. 7**).
- When the needle position is in the desired plane with respect to the dermatotomy and lesion, advance the needle to the proximal edge of the lesion. Continuous observation of the needle is important.
- Before obtaining a sample, ensure that the 2.2-cm excursion of the biopsy needle will not result in injury to the chest wall.
- After the sample is obtained and before removing the needle, scan and take images to document that the needle traversed the lesion (see **Fig. 4**D).
- Five samples are typically obtained if using a 14-gauge throw needle.
- More samples may be useful:
  - o If samples appear fragmented or do not sink when placed in fixative.
  - o In cases of large masses, due to tumor heterogeneity.
  - o In cases where receptor status may be used to guide neoadjuvant therapy.

PLACEMENT OF A RADIOPAQUE MARKER

- Radiopaque marker (Ultraclip; Inrad, Kentwood, MI, USA) placement following sampling is helpful for a variety of reasons (see **Fig. 5**E):
  - o A postprocedure mammogram with biopsy marker in place can confirm concordance between the sonographic and mammographic findings (see **Fig. 2; Fig. 8**D).
  - o A radiopaque marker may be the most obvious or sole imaging evidence denoting the former location of even a large cancer with complete response to neoadjuvant chemotherapy.
  - o A marker placed just posterior to a small or cystic mass before sampling can help subsequent localization of the lesion.
  - o The use of different-shaped markers can help distinguish locations of different lesions undergoing sampling in the same breast.

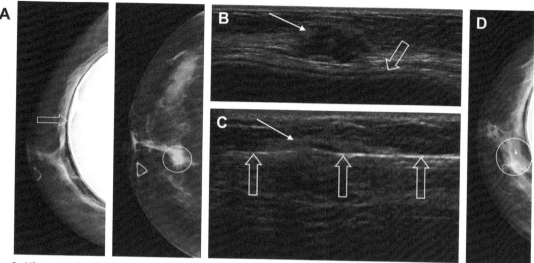

Fig. 8. Ultrasound-guided core-needle biopsy of a palpable suspicious mass in a 42-year-old woman with saline breast implants. (*A*) Craniocaudal view of the right breast shows a palpable mass in the anterior breast, better demonstrated on implant-displaced view (*circle*). There is a saline submuscular implant (*open arrow*). (*B*) Ultrasonography shows a corresponding irregular hypoechoic mass with angular margins and a thin echogenic halo (*arrow*) that is just anterior to the implant (*open arrow*). (*C*) Ultrasound-guided core-needle biopsy was performed using a needle approach (*open arrow*) that is parallel to the implant. The needle traverses the lesion (*arrow*). Histology showed invasive ductal carcinoma. (*D*) Postprocedure mammogram documents a small amount of postbiopsy hemorrhage and clip in the region of the mass (*circle*).

- There are negligible drawbacks to placement of a radiopaque marker; however, It is helpful to inform patients of the following:
  - Titanium markers have minimal interference with breast MR imaging.
  - Markers will not set off airport (or other security) alarms.

FINE-NEEDLE ASPIRATION BIOPSY

In FNAB, the shortest approach to the lesion is used.

- Lidocaine (2%) without epinephrine is injected locally for anesthesia.
- The spinal needle enters the skin at the edge of the transducer and approaches the lesion at an angle of 30° to 45° (see **Fig. 3**).
- The needle is advanced into the lesion, the inner stylet removed, and the needle is moved rapidly back and forth within the lesion. Cells are removed from the lesion using capillary action.
- Typically 2 or 3 passes are made.
- Slides can be prepared immediately by a cytopathology technologist, or the needles can be rinsed in a preservative solution

(Cytolyte; Cytyc Corp., Marlborough, MA, USA) and slides made later.

CHALLENGING CASES
Dense Breast Tissue

- Dense breast tissue can make it difficult to advance the needle.
- A coaxial system with placement of a 12-gauge trocar (TruGuide; Bard, Covington, GA, USA) provides a path to the lesion that can be altered slightly to sample different areas of the lesion without having to traverse dense tissue for each sample.

Implants

- Stereotactic guidance may be an easier approach than ultrasound guidance to a lesion identified mammographically, as the implant can be displaced against the chest wall by the compression paddle.
- However, most lesions can still undergo biopsy using ultrasound guidance (see **Fig. 8**). The presence of an implant increases the need for carefully planning the approach to the lesion.
- A more oblique needle path along the edge of the breast will typically allow the needle path to be parallel to the implant.

Small Lesions

- Lesion visualization can decrease after the first pass or two, or after injection of lidocaine.
- Keeping a small lesion in view during the entire procedure, from injection of lidocaine until the marker is placed, is key.
- Placement of a DVAB device directly posterior to a small lesion and direct visualization while sampling can help to ensure adequate sampling.

Potentially Cystic Lesions

- A very small or very hypoechoic lesion may be difficult to characterize as either cystic or solid (see **Fig. 6**).
- A clip can be placed posterior to the lesion before CNB, which will help subsequent localization of the lesion during sampling and in case surgical biopsy is needed based on the pathology results.

Calcifications

Suspicious calcifications are best sampled using stereotactic guidance.

- While calcifications can often be identified on ultrasonography, be aware that just a small amount of introduced air can obscure calcifications.
- In cases where stereotactic-guided biopsy is not feasible, calcifications can be sampled using ultrasound guidance (see **Fig. 1**).
- DVAB may improve retrieval of calcifications.
- A specimen radiograph should be obtained to confirm adequacy of sampling if the lesion primarily presented as calcifications.
- Placement of a radiopaque marker and postprocedure mammogram can also help to confirm adequate sampling.

Lesions in a Large Breast

Entry at the side of the breast is optimal; however:

- This approach to biopsy a deep lesion in a large breast may result in traversing a long distance.
- Alternatively, a shorter entry point in the anterior breast can be selected.
- To establish a needle path that is parallel to the chest wall, the needle can be used to lift the lesion anteriorly, away from chest wall (**Fig. 9**).

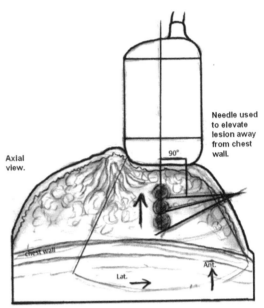

Fig. 9. Core needle biopsy of a deep lesion in a large breast. A needle entry site can be made more anterior on the breast. The lesion can be lifted anteriorly away from the chest wall with the needle to have a path that is still parallel to the chest wall.

Lymph Nodes

A parallel approach is not practical for axillary lymph node core biopsy.

- The medial border of the axilla is defined by the pectoral muscles and the lateral border by the latissimus dorsi muscle, creating a valley where the lymph nodes are often at the deepest aspect.
- A steep approach must therefore be used, similar to that of FNAB.
- Lymph nodes are often immediately anterior to the axillary artery and vein, making the use of long-throw needles difficult.
- Axillary lymph nodes can be sampled using either FNAB or a manually controlled core biopsy needle, such as Temno or Achieve (Cardinal Health, McGraw Park, IL, USA) (**Fig. 10**).
  - FNA of a lymph node is typically all that is needed in the setting of a known or suspected malignancy.
  - Core biopsy is preferred if there is no known or suspected malignancy, as the architecture of the lymph node is needed to make a more useful diagnosis.
  - One or 2 samples may be sent for evaluation by flow cytometry to assess the likelihood of lymphoma, which can be

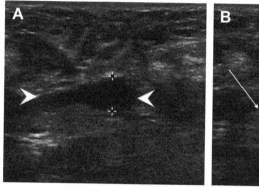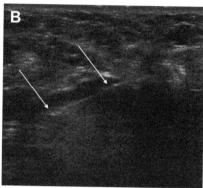

Fig. 10. Ultrasound-guided core-needle biopsy technique for axillary lymph nodes. (*A*) Ultrasonography of a left axillary lymph node (*arrowheads*) in a 41-year-old woman with newly diagnosed invasive breast cancer shows focal cortical thickening suspicious for metastatic disease (*calipers*). (*B*) Ultrasound-guided core-needle biopsy of the suspicious area using a manual-throw needle. The needle is in the open position with the notch centered at the lymph node cortex (*arrows*). The tip of the needle is within the lymph node and will not advance when the sample is obtained. Histology showed metastatic invasive ductal carcinoma.

difficult to diagnose based only on histology of a core biopsy sample.

POSTPROCEDURE EVALUATION

When the procedure is complete:

- Manual pressure is applied over the entire needle path, including the dermatotomy and area of the lesion, for 5 to 10 minutes.
- The dermatotomy can be closed with either a Steri-Strip (3M, St. Paul, MN, USA) or skin adhesive (Dermabond; Ethicon, Inc, Somerville, NJ, USA).
- A postprocedure mammogram can confirm that the lesion sampled corresponds to the mammographic finding of concern (see **Figs. 2** and **8**).
- If the biopsy marker placed after ultrasound-guided biopsy is not present in the mammographic lesion of concern, stereotactic-guided biopsy of the mammographic finding may be necessary (see **Fig. 2**).

COMPLICATIONS AND THEIR MANAGEMENT

Complications from ultrasound-guided biopsy are few.

- The risk of hematoma for patients undergoing ultrasound CNB with a 14-gauge throw needle is approximately 2%.
  - The risk is higher in patients using anticoagulants.

- Infection is very uncommon, and occurs in fewer than 1% of the patients in the authors' practice.
  - When there is concern of postbiopsy infection, treatment with a second-generation cephalosporin, such as cephalexin, is usually adequate.
- In a lactating woman, a milk fistula may develop after CNB. The fistula will not typically resolve until nursing is finished.

RADIOLOGIC-HISTOLOGIC CORRELATION

When biopsy results are received:

- All images from the case should be reviewed for correlation.
- The histology should explain the sonographic (and mammographic or MR imaging) findings.
- If the histology shows malignancy, communication of the results should be given promptly to the patient and referring physician.
- If the histology is benign and concordant, ultrasonography performed after 6 months is helpful to ensure lesion stability.
  - A mammogram can be performed instead of ultrasound if the lesion is well visualized mammographically.
  - If histology returns a specific benign result that is also concordant, such as fibroadenoma, imaging after 1 year can be considered.
- Discordant histology necessitating repeat CNB or surgical biopsy occurs in approximately 3% of cases.

○ When imaging characteristics of the lesion are not explained by the histology, additional sampling by either surgical biopsy or repeat core biopsy should be recommended.

○ Cancer is found at repeat sampling in 24% to 50% of patients. Likewise, if a lesion was assessed as a BI-RADS category 5, surgical biopsy should be considered if a cancer diagnosis is not obtained on CNB histology.

○ Certain histological manifestations found on CNB are considered high risk. Such conditions include atypical ductal hyperplasia (ADH), lobular carcinoma in situ, atypical lobular hyperplasia, radial sclerosing lesion, and papillary lesions.

■ The literature is predominantly based on combined stereotactic (large-gauge) and ultrasound (14-gauge) biopsy, rather than being specific to ultrasound biopsy. The upgrade rate to either ductal carcinoma in situ or invasive cancer is best documented for ADH, at 18% to 50%.

■ Surgical excision should be recommended when core biopsy demonstrates ADH. Management of the remaining lesions is less clear, as these are less common and a wide range of results are reported in the literature.

PATIENT COMMUNICATION

Once the histology is reviewed and a recommendation made, biopsy results can be communicated directly with the patient or to the referring physician, who can relay the results to the patient. Discussion of the results can take place in person or by phone. An addendum to the original biopsy report documents the recommendations and communication of results.

QUALITY

An ongoing quality assurance program should be set up to monitor the outcome of ultrasound-guided breast biopsy. The program should evaluate:

- Positive predictive value
- Benign discordant results
- False-negative outcome
- Complications for the center and by the radiologist
- Available accreditation programs.

SUMMARY

The natural curvature of the breast is used to advantage in ultrasound-guided breast core biopsy. Once mastered, freehand technique is typically the fastest, most accurate method for ultrasound-guided interventions. Entry from the periphery of the breast produces a path that is parallel to the chest wall. Contraindications and complications are few. Challenging cases require additional planning; however, most breast lesions visible on ultrasonography are amenable to ultrasound-guided biopsy. Lesions with discordant biopsy results should undergo repeat sampling, by either percutaneous or excisional biopsy. Results of ultrasound-guided biopsy should be monitored for the center and by each radiologist for quality assurance.

FURTHER READINGS

ACR Practice Guideline for the Performance of Ultrasound-Guided Percutaneous Breast Interventional Procedures. Available at: http://www.acr.org/SecondaryMainMenuCategories/quality_safety/guidelines/breast/us_guided_breast.aspx. Accessed December, 2011. The ACR document lists revision history of: "Revised 2009 (Resolution 29).

American College of Radiology. Breast imaging reporting and data system (BR-RADS). 4th edition. Reston (VA): American College of Radiology; 2003.

Berner A, Davidson B, Sigstad E, et al. Fine-needle aspiration cytology vs. core biopsy in the diagnosis of breast lesions. Diagn Ctyopathol 2003;29(6):344–8.

Brem RF, Lechner MC, Jackman RJ, et al. Lobular neoplasia at percutaneous breast biopsy: variables associated with carcinoma at surgical excision. AJR Am J Roentgenol 2008;190(3):637–41.

Brenner RJ, Jackman RJ, Parker SH, et al. Percutaneous core needle biopsy of radial scars of the breast: when is excision necessary? AJR Am J Roentgenol 2002;179(5):1179–84.

Cavaliere A, Sidoni A, Scheibel M, et al. Biopathologic profile of breast cancer core biopsy: is it always a valid method? Cancer Lett 2005;218(1):117–21.

Crystal P, Koretz M, Shcharynsky S, et al. Accuracy of sonographically guided 14-gauge core-needle biopsy: results of 715 consecutive breast biopsies with at least two-year follow-up of benign lesions. J Clin Ultrasound 2005;33(2):47–52.

Darling MLR, Smith DN, Lester SC, et al. Atypical ductal hyperplasia and ductal carcinoma in situ as revealed by large-core needle breast biopsy: results of surgical excision. AJR Am J Roentgenol 2000; 175(5):1341–6.

Deurloo EE, Tanis PJ, Gilhuijs KG, et al. Reduction in the number of sentinel lymph node procedures by preoperative ultrasonography of the axilla in breast cancer. Eur J Cancer 2004;39(8):1068–73.

Fajardo LL, Pisano ED, Caudry DJ, et al. Radiologist Investigators of the Radiologic Diagnostic Oncology Group V. Stereotactic and sonographic large-core biopsy of nonpalpable breast lesions: results of the Radiologic Diagnostic Oncology Group V study. Acad Radiol 2004;11(3):293–308.

Fishman JE, Milikowski C, Ramsinghani R, et al. US-guided core-needle biopsy of the breast: how many specimens are necessary? Radiology 2003; 226(3):779–82.

Foster MC, Helvie MA, Gregory NE, et al. Lobular carcinoma in situ or atypical lobular hyperplasia at core-needle biopsy: is excisional biopsy necessary? Radiology 2004;231(3):813–9.

Harvey JA, Cohen MA, Brenin DR, et al. Breaking bad news: a primer for radiologists in breast imaging. J Am Coll Radiol 2007;4(11):800–8.

Jackman RJ, Burbank F, Parker SH, et al. Atypical ductal hyperplasia diagnosed at stereotactic breast biopsy: improved reliability with 14-gauge, directional, vacuum-assisted biopsy. Radiology 1997;204(2): 485–8.

Jackman RJ, Nowels KW, Shepard MJ, et al. Stereotaxic large-core needle biopsy of 450 nonpalpable breast lesions with surgical correlation in lesions with cancer or atypical hyperplasia. Radiology 1994; 193(1):91–5.

Lannin DR, Ponn T, Andrejeva L, et al. Should all breast cancers be diagnosed by needle biopsy? Am J Surg 2006;192(4):450–4.

Liberman L, Drotman M, Morris EA, et al. Imaging-histologic discordance at percutaneous breast biopsy. Cancer 2000;89(12):2538–46.

Liberman L, Ernberg LA, Heerdt A, et al. Palpable breast masses: is there a role for percutaneous imaging-guided core biopsy? AJR Am J Roentgenol 2000; 175(3):779–87.

Liberman L, Goodstine SL, Dershaw DD, et al. One operation after percutaneous diagnosis of nonpalpable breast cancer: frequency and associated factors. AJR Am J Roentgenol 2002;178(3): 673–9.

Liberman L. Centennial dissertation. Percutaneous image-guided core breast biopsy: state of the art at the millennium. AJR Am J Roentgenol 2000; 174:1191–9.

Melotti MK, Berg WA. Core needle breast biopsy in patients undergoing anticoagulation therapy: preliminary results. AJR Am J Roentgenol 2000; 174(1):245–9.

Nath ME, Robinson TM, Tobon H, et al. Automated large-core needle biopsy of surgically removed breast lesions: comparison of samples obtained with 14-, 16-, and 18-gauge needles. Radiology 1995; 197(3):739–42.

Parker SH, Burbank F, Jackman RJ, et al. Percutaneous large-core breast biopsy: a multi-institutional study. Radiology 1994;193(2):359–64.

Philpotts LE, Hooley RJ, Lee CH. Comparison of automated versus vacuum-assisted biopsy methods for sonographically guided core biopsy of the breast. AJR Am J Roentgenol 2003;180(2):347–51.

Pisano ED, Fajardo LL, Caudry DJ, et al. Fine-needle aspiration biopsy of nonpalpable breast lesions in a multicenter clinical trial: results from the radiologic diagnostic oncology group V. Radiology 2001; 219(3):785–92.

Schackmuth EM, Harlow CL, Norton LW. Milk fistula: a complication after core breast biopsy. AJR Am J Roentgenol 1993;161(5):961–2.

Shin HJ, Kim HH, Kim SM, et al. Papillary lesions of the breast diagnosed at percutaneous sonographically guided biopsy: comparison of sonographic features and biopsy methods. AJR Am J Roentgenol 2008; 190(3):630–6.

Simon JR, Kalbhen CL, Cooper RA, et al. Accuracy and complication rates of US-guided vacuum-assisted core breast biopsy: initial results. Radiology 2000; 215(3):694–7.

Soo MS, Baker JA, Rosen EL. Sonographic detection and sonographically guided biopsy of breast microcalcifications. AJR Am J Roentgenol 2003;180(4):941–8.

Youk JH, Kim EK, Kim MJ, et al. Sonographically guided 14-gauge core needle biopsy of breast masses: a review of 2,420 cases with long-term follow-up. AJR Am J Roentgenol 2008;190(1):202–7.

Ultrasound-Guided Procedures in Obstetrics

Christian A. Chisholm, MD*, James E. Ferguson II, MD, MBA

KEYWORDS

- Ultrasound • Obstetrics • Diagnosis • Complications

KEY POINTS

- Amniocentesis and chorionic villus sampling are the most common techniques for obtaining a prenatal karyotype on a fetus at risk; in appropriately-trained hands, either can be performed with an acceptably low risk of complications.
- Ultrasound guidance is used for nearly all invasive diagnostic procedures in obstetrics, and seems to improve the odds for a successful procedure, but may not reduce the risk of procedure-related pregnancy loss.
- Ultrasound guidance is essential for fetal therapeutic interventions such as fetal blood transfusion, vesicoamniotic shunt placement, and thoracentesis.

INTRODUCTION

Ultrasound is used to provide guidance for invasive procedures during pregnancy because it is the primary imaging modality used in the antenatal period. In addition to the documented safety of ultrasound and the absence of ionizing radiation exposure to the fetus, ultrasound offers the unique advantage of real-time imaging, allowing continuous ultrasound monitoring of invasive diagnostic procedures. This quality of ultrasound monitoring allowed the initial development and further refinement of fetal therapeutic procedures.

Amniocentesis was the first procedure performed for invasive fetal diagnosis, for Rh disease in the late 1950s, and for genetic diagnosis in the late 1960s. Although preprocedure mapping of an amniotic fluid pocket was possible using static scanning, real-time ultrasound guidance was not introduced until the 1980s. With this advance came the opportunity to introduce additional diagnostic techniques including chorionic villus sampling, fetal blood sampling, and aspiration of fetal urine to assess fetal renal function. Although intrauterine fetal transfusion was the earliest fetal therapeutic intervention (with intraperitoneal transfusion again dating to the era before ultrasound guidance was available), several additional therapeutic interventions for the fetus have been developed in the modern era.

In most centers, genetic counseling is an integral part of a patient's decision to undergo invasive prenatal diagnosis testing, whether by amniocentesis or chorionic villus sampling. A genetic counseling encounter allows the opportunity to gather a detailed family history and to provide counseling regarding the relative risks of invasive diagnostic testing and noninvasive screening. The core principle of genetic counseling is its nondirective nature, in which the aim is to provide adequate information to facilitate patient decision making.

AMNIOCENTESIS

There are several current indications for amniocentesis (**Box 1**). Amniocentesis was first proposed as a routine consideration for women older than 35 years in the late 1970s by the National Institutes of Health. The threshold of age 35 years, which persists today in the International Classification

Disclosures: None.
Department of Obstetrics and Gynecology, The University of Virginia, PO Box 800712, Charlottesville, VA 22908, USA
* Corresponding author.
E-mail address: CAC2U@Virginia.edu

Ultrasound Clin 7 (2012) 325–335
doi:10.1016/j.cult.2012.03.006

> **Box 1**
> **Indications for amniocentesis**
>
> Advanced maternal age
>
> Abnormal genetic screening
>
> - First-trimester screening
> - Second-trimester maternal serum screening
>
> Family history of genetic disorder
>
> - Prior child with fetal aneuploidy or other genetic disorder
> - Other family history of a disorder for which prenatal diagnosis by DNA analysis is available
>
> Abnormal ultrasound findings
>
> Increased maternal serum α-fetoprotein
>
> Red cell or platelet alloimmunization
>
> Fetal lung maturity testing
>
> Evaluation for intra-amniotic infection
>
> Evaluation for rupture of fetal membranes (dye test)
>
> Therapeutic reduction of amniotic fluid volume for symptomatic hydramnios

of Diseases (ICD-10) diagnosis code for advanced maternal age, was selected in recognition of epidemiologic data showing a higher risk for fetal Down syndrome in women more than 35 years old compared with those age 30 to 34 years. This age threshold to offer amniocentesis also took into account the relative availability of trained operators and cytogenetic laboratories, and made an attempt to balance the risk of an abnormal finding against the risk of a procedure-related loss. This threshold criterion is still used as the basis for establishing criteria to offer invasive testing with other forms of screening (1:270 risk or higher of Down syndrome).[1]

However, the risk of fetal aneuploidy is a continuous variable that increases with maternal age, therefore the use of maternal age as the sole screening criterion for fetal aneuploidy has major limitations. It is widely recognized that most (70%–80%) aneuploid conceptions occur in women less than 35 years old.

A substantial goal of new advances in prenatal diagnosis is the reduction in procedure-related pregnancy losses, in conjunction with enhanced detection rates of fetal aneuploidy. Noninvasive screening tests such as first-trimester genetic screening or second-trimester maternal serum screening offer women less than 35 years old the opportunity to be identified as having an increased risk for fetal Down syndrome and thus the option to pursue invasive diagnostic testing. Screening tests also present the opportunity for women more than 35 years old to undergo screening before making a decision about invasive diagnostic testing, and perhaps opt out of diagnostic testing (and its attendant risk) if their likelihood of aneuploidy after screening is reduced. An important element of counseling women more than 35 years old regarding screening is a discussion of the false-negative and false-positive rates associated with screening. The recent development of noninvasive techniques to identify alterations in the rate of single-nucleotide polymorphisms (SNPs) in maternal blood raises the possibility of identifying fetal Down syndrome and other fetal aneuploidies with high precision and few false-positives by noninvasive means.

As new noninvasive tests become commercially available, the indications for invasive prenatal diagnosis will decrease, and the number of procedures being performed will decrease in parallel. The rate of procedure-related loss is also expected to decrease once this development becomes a reality. A downward trend over time in procedure volumes has already been reported by some investigators.[2,3] As the number of women with an indication for prenatal diagnostic testing declines, it will be essential for specialists in maternal-fetal medicine and perinatal genetics to continue to receive training and maintain their skills in invasive prenatal diagnostic procedures, which have largely become the domain of subspecialists, and are rarely performed currently by general obstetrician-gynecologists or by radiologists.

Technique

In the modern era, continuous ultrasound monitoring/guidance of amniocentesis is considered essential. The use of ultrasound allows continuous guidance and visualization of the needle into the amniotic fluid within the gestational sac, as well as identification of fetal movements and change in fetal position, either of which could result in fetal injury if the needle were inserted without ultrasound visualization. Ultrasound guidance allows the identification of membrane tenting, a possible explanation for absence of fluid return. Amniocentesis studies published during the era of continuous ultrasound guidance have not shown a reduction in the pregnancy loss rate attributable to amniocentesis compared with studies of procedures performed before ultrasound guidance was routine, although they have shown a reduction in the rate of obtaining bloody amniotic fluid and the number of needle insertions required to obtain a fluid sample. Fetal injury at the time of amniocentesis is rare. After patient counseling is complete and informed consent has been obtained, the abdomen is prepared with an antiseptic solution; we prefer the use of chlorhexidine-alcohol, which is allowed to dry on the abdomen before performing the procedure. Povidone-iodine solution is an acceptable alternative. Coupling gel is applied to the ultrasound transducer, which is inserted into a sterile probe cover or sterile glove, and sterile coupling gel is applied to the abdomen. Under real-time ultrasonography, an appropriate needle insertion site is selected. The ideal insertion site is a pocket of amniotic fluid that is free of fetal parts and does not require traversing the placenta. In cases in which the placenta is implanted anteriorly, placental penetration may be unavoidable; however, ultrasound guidance makes it possible to avoid the edges of the placenta as well as the central area where the umbilical cord inserts and, ideally, to avoid traversing large vessels on the placental surface. Color Doppler may aid in identifying these vessels. These precautions reduce the likelihood of a bloody sample. We use a 22-gauge spinal needle, selecting one with a modified echogenic tip in obese women or when oligohydramnios is present to enhance visualization of the needle tip. Some operators prefer a 20-gauge needle. The needle is inserted along the plane of the transducer (coplanar), with or without the use of a needle guide, to allow visualization of the needle path. It is advanced through the myometrium (**Fig. 1**) and into the amniotic sac, where the stylet is withdrawn. The usual quantity of amniotic fluid withdrawn for genetic analysis is 20 to 30 mL, with the first 1 to 2 mL either discarded or used for α-fetoprotein determination, to avoid potential contamination of the amniotic fluid cell culture with maternal cells on the needle tip from the process of insertion. After needle removal, fetal

heart rate is confirmed and the site of myometrial or placental penetration is visualized to ensure there is no bleeding. Rh immune globulin is administered if the woman is Rh negative and unsensitized. She is advised to avoid strenuous activity for 1 to 2 days after the procedure, to anticipate mild cramping for several hours, and to report vaginal leakage of watery amniotic fluid, vaginal bleeding, malodorous vaginal discharge, lower abdominal tenderness, or fever. Depending on the test requested, preliminary cytogenetic results may be available in as little as 1 to 2 days if fluorescent in-situ hybridization techniques are used, or may take as long as 2 to 3 weeks with conventional culture techniques or if DNA analysis is to be performed.

In the case of multiple gestations, each amniotic sac is sampled separately. Most operators instill 1 to 2 mL of indigo carmine dye after withdrawing the amniotic fluid sample from the first and each subsequent fetus as an additional measure to be certain that each fetus is sampled separately. If, during the second needle insertion into the sac of the other fetus in twins, the fluid obtained is blue, then the first fetus has been sampled twice and reinsertion is necessary to sample the second. Some operators have advocated a single-needle insertion technique, with intentional penetration of the intertwin membrane to sample the second fetus. Neither approach has been subjected to rigorous study, although we prefer to sample each sac separately.

Complications

The greatest concern for most couples deciding whether to undergo amniocentesis is the likelihood of fetal loss. The maternal age threshold and screening cutoff of age 35 years, or 1 in 270 risk of Down syndrome, has been retained in part because it is thought to reflect a balance between the likelihood of abnormal findings and the risk of a procedure-related loss. Historically, most centers have counseled their couples that the risk of miscarriage after amniocentesis is up to 0.5% (unless they have center-specific data on which to base their counseling).

The first reports describing the rate of amniocentesis-related pregnancy loss came from before the era of high-resolution real-time ultrasound that could be used for guidance. In a United States study of 2000 women, fetal loss between the time of the procedure and delivery occurred in 3.5% of women compared with 3.2% of controls, a nonsignificant difference.[4] A similar rate of 3.2% without a control group was reported in a Canadian study.[5] Subsequently, a Danish

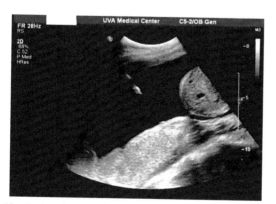

Fig. 1. Amniocentesis needle in place.

study published in 1986 showed a miscarriage rate of 1.7% in the amniocentesis group compared with 0.7% in controls (P<.01), in a highly selected population.[6] More recent reports have questioned the association between amniocentesis and an increased risk of pregnancy loss. In a study from Thailand published in 1998 involving 2256 women undergoing amniocentesis with matched controls, no difference was found in the rate of spontaneous abortion after amniocentesis (1.8%) versus controls (1.4%), (P>.05). No other complication seemed to be increased in the amniocentesis group.[7] A more recent Thai study[8] showed similar results in a cohort of 5051 pregnant women referred for prenatal counseling and followed prospectively, with subsequent comparison of those who underwent amniocentesis with those who declined. There were no differences in fetal loss rates before 24 weeks, before 28 weeks, or in the rate of preterm delivery. Towner and colleagues[9] reported similar results in a cohort of more than 32,000 women from the California State Maternal Serum Screening Program, with a miscarriage rate that was no different between women who chose amniocentesis and those who did not. In addition, Odibo and colleagues[10] reported on a 16-year experience at a single center encompassing more than 11,000 women undergoing amniocentesis and nearly 40,000 women in the same gestational period who did not undergo a diagnostic procedure. A significant difference between this study and the others mentioned earlier is that the control group represented an unselected population of women having ultrasound at the same gestational age as those undergoing amniocentesis, rather than age-matched controls who were referred for, but did not undergo, amniocentesis. The controls had a lower mean maternal age and lower proportion of women more than 35 years of age, as well as other risk factors such as prior family history of genetic disorders. In this study, the fetal loss rate before 24 weeks' gestation was 0.97% for the amniocentesis group and 0.84% for the group not undergoing a procedure, suggesting that the fetal loss rate before 24 weeks that was attributable to amniocentesis was 0.13%, or 1 in 769 procedures. This result represents a substantially lower risk than that typically used for prenatal diagnosis counseling.

An analysis of these reports suggests that when performed at the traditional gestational range of 16 to 20 weeks, the risk of miscarriage associated with amniocentesis is 0.5% or less, allowing women to make an informed decision understanding the risk of the procedure and weighing it against her estimated risk for diagnosis of a fetal abnormality, as well as her desire to receive diagnostic information before the birth of her child.

Less clear is the miscarriage rate attributable to amniocentesis in a twin gestation. In a recently published study from Greece, the investigators compared the outcomes of 120 women undergoing amniocentesis in a twin gestation with 6150 undergoing amniocentesis in a singleton gestation, with advanced maternal age being the most common indication for the procedure. In this study, the women with twin pregnancies were statistically of lower parity and more likely to have become pregnant as a result of in vitro fertilization. They reported a miscarriage rate of 0.24% for singletons and 0% in twins with miscarriage defined as pregnancy loss before 24 weeks; this difference was not statistically significant.[11] Conversely, Cahill and colleagues[12] reported the outcomes of twin pregnancies undergoing and not undergoing amniocentesis at Washington University, and showed a 3.2% rate of pregnancy loss in those having an amniocentesis compared with 1.4% in those who did not; they concluded that the attributable risk of fetal loss in twin pregnancies undergoing amniocentesis was 1.8%. This study has the same potential limitations as the Odibo and colleagues[10] study of amniocentesis in singletons, including younger maternal age and mean gravidity in women not having an amniocentesis.[12] Given these reports, it may be advisable to counsel women undergoing amniocentesis with twins of the potential of a higher rate of pregnancy loss than for amniocentesis in singletons. Counseling women with twins is made more complicated by the potential for discordant karyotypic results in dizygotic twins and the challenging management decisions in a twin pregnancy with 1 normal and 1 abnormal fetus.

Early gestational age at amniocentesis has been consistently implicated as a risk factor for an increased rate of pregnancy loss. In several studies in which amniocentesis was performed as early as 11 to 13 weeks' gestation as an alternative to a chorionic villus sampling, the miscarriage rate was reported to be as much as 4 times higher compared with women undergoing amniocentesis in the traditional gestational age range of 16 to 20 weeks.[13–15] Likewise, the occurrence of bloody amniotic fluid is increased significantly. Early amniocentesis is mentioned here only for perspective, in that it is rarely offered clinically, particularly with the availability of more data regarding the safety of chorionic villus sampling (discussed later).

Other complications of amniocentesis are less common and include amniotic fluid leakage and vaginal bleeding. In most cases, these are transient events that cease spontaneously. The occurrence of amniotic fluid leakage that results in oligohydramnios is of greater concern because the presence of a sufficient quantity of amniotic fluid is essential for fetal lung development. Several investigators have proposed techniques for ultrasound-guided intra-amniotic instillation of thrombogenic substrate to serve as a patch over the site of apparent rupture, with variable success.[16] Epidemiologic data suggest the possibility of a mild increase in the risk of congenital talipes equinovarus (club foot) in women undergoing amniocentesis compared with those who do not,[17] as well as for placental abruption.[18]

In summary, women undergoing second-trimester amniocentesis may be informed of a low risk of complications, with a miscarriage risk not exceeding 0.5% for singleton pregnancies, but potentially higher for twin gestations. As always, the most important considerations in assuring the safest possible execution of the procedure include adherence to appropriate indications for the procedure, the presence of a skilled operator, and the use of ultrasound guidance.

CHORIONIC VILLUS SAMPLING

Chorionic villus sampling (CVS) is an ultrasound-guided biopsy of the chorion frondosum of the developing placenta. Indications for CVS are listed in **Box 2**. Retrieval of chorionic villi allows isolation of cells from the rapidly dividing and highly cellular cytotrophoblast for karyotype analysis. CVS is most commonly performed between 10 and 13 weeks' gestation by the transcervical route. Transabdominal procedures can be performed at any

---

Box 2
Indications for CVS

Advanced maternal age

Abnormal first-trimester screening

Family history of genetic disorder

- Prior child with fetal aneuploidy or other genetic disorder

Other family history of a disorder for which prenatal diagnosis by DNA analysis is available

Contraindications:

Maternal red cell alloimmunization

Possibly maternal chronic viral infection (human immunodeficiency virus, hepatitis)

Active infection at site of needle or catheter placement

---

gestational age after 10 weeks and provide an alternative means of obtaining a karyotype in pregnancies affected by severe oligohydramnios. Ultrasound guidance for CVS is essential for localization of the placenta and assurance of aspiration of an adequate tissue sample. Most often, the approach to CVS is dictated by operator preference and experience along with patient choice; however, there are certain circumstances in which only 1 approach is appropriate, and therefore operators should remain proficient in both techniques. A posterior placenta is typically only accessible by transcervical CVS unless the uterus is also sharply anteverted. A fundal placenta is typically only accessible transabdominally. Transabdominal sampling is more likely to be used in multifetal gestations to avoid contamination of one cell culture with another, which could occur as a result of sampling multiple placentas through the cervix.

Technique

Both approaches are preceded by a complete transabdominal ultrasound examination including placental localization, assessment of uterine position, and a basic assessment of fetal well-being including gestational age. Neither should be attempted if infection is present on the maternal abdomen in the area of needle insertion, or in the cervix in the case of a transcervical approach. The woman maintains a full bladder until the procedure is completed; the bladder provides an essential sonographic window for adequate imaging during the procedure. For transcervical procedures, the woman assumes a dorsal lithotomy position, the external genitalia may be prepared with povidone-iodine solution, and a vaginal speculum is inserted. The cervix and vaginal walls are prepared with additional povidone-iodine and the operator changes gloves before starting the procedure. The transcervical CVS catheter is a flexible polyethylene catheter over a malleable aluminum obturator with a blunt tip. The operator shapes the catheter to assume the curvature of the cervical canal and uterus and guides the catheter tip into the placenta. The sonographer follows advancement of the tip past the internal cervical os until it is placed into a long axis of the placenta, ideally about midway through the thickness (**Fig. 2**). The obturator is removed, and a 10-mL syringe containing 5 mL of nutrient medium is attached. Negative pressure is applied while the catheter is withdrawn. Visual inspection of the sample typically allows confirmation of the presence of an adequate sample of chorionic villi (typically 20–30 mg). In some

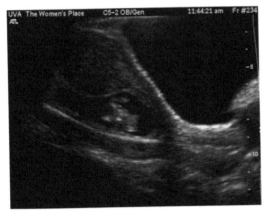

Fig. 2. CVS catheter in place in a posterior placenta.

cases, examination under a dissecting microscope is necessary to assure an adequate sample size before the procedure is completed. A second sample may be performed if the first sample size is small. It is important that only chorionic villi (representing fetal tissue) are cultured rather than decidual cells (maternal tissue), because they can occasionally be aspirated.

Transabdominal CVS is preceded by sterile abdominal preparation with either povidone-iodine or chlorhexidine-alcohol. A coplanar needle insertion technique similar to a transabdominal amniocentesis is used, and a 19-gauge or 20-gauge needle is used. Once the needle has been placed into a long axis of the placenta, many operators use a pistol grip for the syringe, and villi are then aspirated into the syringe similarly to the transcervical technique. A to-and-fro motion of the needle tip within the placenta is made several times to ensure removal of an adequate number of villi because the needle diameter is smaller than the transcervical CVS catheter. Again, the sample is inspected for adequacy.

After either approach, fetal heart tones are verified and Rh immune globulin administered if the woman is Rh negative. She is instructed to avoid strenuous activities for 24 to 48 hours and to alert her provider if she experiences vaginal bleeding in excess of spotting, watery discharge, severe cramping, lower abdominal tenderness, or fever. Results from direct analysis of mitotic figures in cytotrophoblast cells may be available in as soon as 2 days, with a full culture leading to results in 8 to 14 days. The time to achieve results is, in part, related to the size of the sample (milligrams of villi).

Complications

When considering complications of CVS, it is important to carefully review the reports of procedure-related loss rates and to put those into the context of the gestational age at which chorionic villus sampling is performed. Because this procedure is typically performed at 10 to 13 weeks of gestation, the background rate of pregnancy loss (the rate of pregnancy loss irrespective of whether an invasive procedure is performed) is higher compared with amniocentesis at 15 to 18 weeks. This difference is borne out in most reports comparing the loss rates of these 2 procedures. It is important to provide reasonable estimations of the risk of loss to patients because they make decisions about which procedure they wish to pursue based in part on the estimated likelihood of pregnancy loss related to the procedure, as well as their desire to have results as early in the pregnancy as possible. The typical loss rate described for CVS is 0.5% to 1%, or 1 in 200 to 1 in 100 procedures.[19]

Several recent publications have reported on the rates of pregnancy loss for CVS compared with amniocentesis. Mujezinovic and Alfirevic[20] published a systematic review of 16 studies of transabdominal CVS and 29 studies of amniocentesis. Each of the included studies reported on the outcomes of at least 100 procedures. They reported on pregnancy loss rates within 14 days of the procedure by 24 weeks' gestation, and total pregnancy loss. The rates for amniocentesis were 0.6%, 0.9%, and 1.9% respectively. In comparison, the rates for CVS were 0.7%, 1.3%, and 2%. These differences were not statistically significant.[20] The investigators commented that the major limitation of the studies included in this systematic review was the lack of properly selected controls. Caughey and colleagues[21] reported in 2006 on the comparative experience of nearly 10,000 CVS procedures and 30,000 amniocentesis procedures at a single center. The rate of pregnancy loss for both procedures decreased with time and the difference in loss rate between procedures became nonsignificant after 1993.

More recently, Tabor and colleagues[2] in 2009 reported a national registry study over a 10-year period in Denmark including 32,852 amniocentesis and 31, 355 transabdominal CVS procedures. The loss rates were 1.4% and 1.9% respectively when a procedure-related loss was defined as a miscarriage or intrauterine fetal death before 24 weeks' gestation.[2] These experienced investigators concluded that the difference in loss rate between the procedures was possibly attributable to the gestational age difference at the time the procedures were performed. They also observed that the loss rates were lower in centers performing a higher volume of procedures during the study period. In addition, Odibo and colleagues[22] reported a cohort of 5243 women undergoing CVS at a single center over 16 years, and compared them with a control group of women having an ultrasound showing a viable fetus at the same gestational age. The control group was not comparable with the CVS group in that the control women were younger, had their ultrasound at a later gestational age, were more likely to be white, and had experienced fewer prior miscarriages. They did not detect a difference in the fetal loss rate between these groups.

There have been few studies addressing the difference in loss rate attributable to transabdominal versus transcervical CVS. Jackson and colleagues[23] reported the results of a trial of 3999 women randomly assigned to undergo transabdominal or transcervical CVS. The mean gestational age at the time of procedure in both groups was 10.9 weeks, and 80% of procedures in both groups were performed at 10 or 11 weeks. No differences were seen in loss rate or live birth rate by route. In another report, Silver and colleagues[24] described a series of more than 1000 CVS procedures performed between 9 and 12 weeks' gestation, and reported a loss rate for transcervical CVS of 5.2% compared with 2.9% for transabdominal CVS. This apparent difference in loss rate did not reach statistical significance.

No discussion of CVS is complete without mention of the controversy surrounding limb reduction defects. In 1991, Firth and colleagues[25] reported that, among 289 women undergoing CVS at less than 66 days' gestation (approximately 9.5 weeks), there were 5 cases of severe limb abnormalities and oromandibular-limb hypogenesis syndrome. Although this finding had not been reported by other observers, approximately 1 year later, Burton and colleagues[26] reported 4 cases of minor limb reduction defects from the first 500 CVS procedures performed in a newly established CVS program. The CVS procedures in this series were all performed after 10 weeks' gestation. In this cohort, the CVS-related pregnancy loss rate was 8% compared with the 1% to 2% reported by most other centers. There was a significant subsequent reduction in patient interest in CVS because of concerns about limb reduction abnormalities. However, large population-based registries have failed to substantiate concerns about limb reduction abnormalities for CVS performed after 10 weeks' gestation. The World Health Organization registry of 138,996 prospectively ascertained cases of CVS included 77 fetuses with limb reduction defects. This finding corresponded with an incidence of limb reduction defects in

CVS-exposed pregnancies of 5.2 to 5.7 per 10,000, which compared favorably with the background rate of limb reduction abnormalities in the population of 4.8 to 5.97 per 10,000. The authors of these reports concluded that CVS after 10 weeks' gestation was not a risk factor for fetal limb reduction defects.[27,28]

The final complication attributable to CVS is that of either not obtaining results or obtaining nondiagnostic results. Culture failure is reported to occur in up to 1% of CVS samplings and the likelihood of culture seems to be inversely related to the sample size. In addition, mosaicism (the presence of 2 distinct cell lines in the cell culture, usually in substantially different proportions) is found in 1.3% of CVS cases.[29] Although mosaicism is nearly always confined to the placenta, amniocentesis or other diagnostic techniques are necessary to exclude the unlikely possibility that the mosaicism also affects fetal tissue rather than simply the placenta.

FETAL BLOOD SAMPLING

CVS is exclusively a diagnostic procedure, and nearly all amniocentesis procedures are performed for diagnostic purposes as well. Fetal blood sampling serves as a diagnostic tool but also provides access for fetal therapeutic interventions by transfusion of blood products and administration of pharmacologic agents and holds promise for other future interventions such as gene therapy. Indications for fetal blood sampling are listed in **Box 3**. Because of the technically challenging nature of fetal blood sampling, as well as the small number of indications, it is essential that this procedure be performed by individuals with current knowledge in the techniques and contraindications.

Box 3
Indications for fetal blood sampling

Fetal karyotyping (when a rapid karyotype is needed or when a karyotype cannot be obtained by amniocentesis caused by oligohydramnios)

Fetus at risk for genetic disorder for which prenatal diagnosis by DNA analysis is available

Fetus at risk for anemia or thrombocytopenia

Suspected or known fetal infection (parvovirus, cytomegalovirus, toxoplasma)

Determination of fetal acid-base status (uncommonly performed)

Technique

Fetal blood sampling can be performed as early as 20 to 22 weeks of gestation (potentially earlier in skilled hands), and as late as term; the upper gestational age limit is often determined when a threshold is reached at which the risk of a complication of the procedure is thought to exceed the risks to the fetus of preterm delivery, often approximately 34 weeks. When this procedure is being performed before fetal viability, the ambulatory setting is appropriate; however, when fetal blood sampling (with or without transfusion) is to be performed at a gestational age when the fetus is potentially viable ex utero, and when intervention by emergency cesarean would be considered in the event of a complication of the procedure, then it is prudent to do so in an inpatient setting, most frequently in the labor and delivery unit where an emergency cesarean is readily available.

Before performing the procedure, a detailed ultrasound examination is performed with special attention to the location of the placenta and the placental cord insertion site. After obtaining informed consent and thoroughly preparing the abdomen with either chlorhexidine-alcohol or povidone-iodine, the procedure is initiated. With the transabdominal ultrasound transducer in a sterile sleeve, an appropriate needle insertion site is selected. The most common access points for fetal blood sampling and or transfusion are the placental insertion of the umbilical cord, the intrahepatic portion of the fetal umbilical vein, or a free loop of umbilical cord. The placental insertion site is particularly favored with an anterior or fundal placenta and is also a good choice because of its relative stability (**Fig. 3**). However, traversing the placenta usually results in a small amount of fetomaternal transfusion and, if the indication for the fetal blood sampling is alloimmunization, this may expose the mother to additional fetal blood and accelerate the immune response. A free loop of umbilical cord is the least stable option, because fetal movements may dislodge the needle.

Local anesthetic is administered at the needle insertion site and a 22-gauge spinal needle is inserted under continuous ultrasound guidance. The required skill level of the sonographer providing guidance for fetal blood sampling is substantially higher than that required for amniocentesis. The target for the needle insertion is smaller and therefore the margin of error is narrower. A suitable amniotic fluid pocket for amniocentesis is generally 2 × 2 cm or larger, making it easier for the sonographer to adjust the transducer to identify the needle. In the case of fetal blood sampling, the sonographer must maintain continuous visualization of the umbilical vein at the proposed insertion site and assist the operator in redirection of the needle until it reaches the target. Confirmation of umbilical vein puncture is obtained by removing the stylet from the needle, attaching a heparinized 1-mL syringe, and obtaining blood return (**Fig. 4**). At the conclusion of the procedure, the stylet is replaced, the needle is withdrawn, and fetal heart motion is confirmed. The puncture site of the umbilical vein is observed to ensure that the bleeding stops. This usually occurs in less than 30 seconds. For nonimmunized Rh-negative patients, Rh immune globulin is administered and, if the fetus is at a potentially viable gestational age, fetal monitoring is initiated for several hours to assure fetal well-being after the procedure.

Most operators performing fetal blood transfusion perform the transfusion at the same setting as the diagnostic fetal blood sampling, rather than performing 1 procedure to diagnose fetal anemia and a second to treat the anemia with transfusion. This method represents a logical risk-reduction strategy because each separate procedure has a procedure-related loss rate of

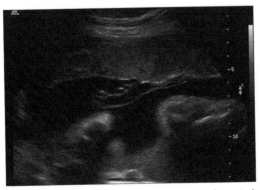

Fig. 3. Placental cord insertion to anterior placenta in advance of fetal blood sampling.

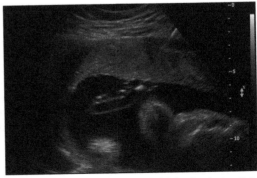

Fig. 4. Needle in lumen of umbilical vein during fetal blood sampling.

approximately 1%. However, this requires a coordinated effort between the perinatal team and the blood bank to have appropriately cross-matched, CMV-negative, irradiated, highly packed (hematocrit 75%) red blood cells available at the initiation of the procedure, and to have precalculated the appropriate volume to be transfused based on the sonographic estimated fetal weight, the estimated fetal placental blood volume, and hypothetical starting hematocrit. Fetal neuromuscular blockade with pancuronium or vecuronium may be used for transfusion procedures because of their increased duration, but may not be necessary for diagnostic-only fetal blood sampling. Neuromuscular blockade may also not be necessary if the needle insertion does not pass through the amniotic sac. When fetal blood sampling and/or transfusion is being performed for platelet alloimmunization, it is critically important to have cross-matched platelets available. Streaming of blood from the needle insertion site after fetal blood sampling is common, occurring in 40% to 50% of cases and typically lasting less than 60 seconds. However, in a fetus with severe alloimmune thrombocytopenia, the normal hemostatic mechanisms are impaired and blood loss from the needle puncture site can be substantial unless platelets are transfused.

Complications

The pregnancy loss rate for fetal blood sampling has generally been reported to range from 1% to 3%.[30,31] The likelihood for loss is related to the experience of the operator, the indications for the procedure, the technique used, and the gestational age. Because of this high loss rate, many operators place an upper gestational age limit at which they would no longer perform fetal blood sampling but would rather move to delivery in a fetus with an indication for fetal blood sampling. This gestational age is often set at approximately 34 weeks, when the risk to the fetus of complications or preterm may be lower than the risk of complications from the procedure. Ghidini and colleagues[32] reported a fetal loss rate of 2.7% in low-risk fetuses undergoing fetal blood sampling, defining low risk as those fetuses in which no abnormality was found at the time of the procedure. Among the high-risk fetuses, which included those with chromosomal abnormalities, severe fetal growth restriction, fetal infections, and fetal hydrops, the loss rate was substantially higher at 9.4%.

OTHER ULTRASOUND-GUIDED PROCEDURES

Early success of fetal blood transfusion as a therapeutic intervention has led to the promise of other interventions to improve pregnancy outcome and avoid preterm delivery. A wide variety of ultrasound-guided fetal interventions have been reported with variable success. For example, fetal pleural effusions can be drained by ultrasound-guided needle placement into the fetal thorax, allowing expansion of the lung (**Fig. 5**). Although hypothetically this reduces the likelihood of pulmonary hypoplasia, there is a lack of adequate prospective studies to support this contention. In a similar manner, fetal ascites could be aspirated for both diagnostic and therapeutic purposes. Fetal skin and muscle biopsy have been described for the diagnosis of specific disorders, such a congenital ichthyosis and muscular dystrophy.

Perhaps the most well established ultrasound-guided fetal therapeutic procedure after fetal blood transfusion is vesicoamniotic shunting for fetuses with bladder outlet obstruction (posterior urethral valves, urethral atresia). A fetus with bladder outlet obstruction may be diagnosed early in pregnancy by the findings of a massively distended urinary bladder and decreased or absent amniotic fluid. Although the urinary obstruction ultimately leads to kidney damage, most untreated fetuses with bladder outlet obstruction die from pulmonary hypoplasia caused by the absence of amniotic fluid to facilitate normal lung development. The purpose of vesicoamniotic shunting is to bypass the obstructed urethra and allow fetal urine to drain through a shunt that traverses the bladder wall and the anterior abdominal wall into the amniotic sac to restore normal amniotic fluid volume.[33] Before shunting, fetal urine is aspirated under ultrasound guidance for analysis of urine electrolytes to assess prognosis for long-term renal function. Vesicoamniotic shunting has met with fairly consistent success and is generally accepted in fetal medicine as an appropriate therapeutic intervention for fetuses with bladder outlet

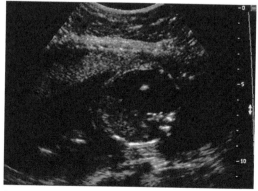

Fig. 5. Needle placement in fetal chest for diagnostic fetal thoracentesis.

obstruction, although it may ultimately be replaced by laparoscopically guided, minimally invasive laser ablation of the posterior urethral valves. A discussion of that procedure as well as other diagnostic or therapeutic techniques is beyond the scope of this article.

REFERENCES

1. Wapner RJ, Jenkins TM, Khalek N. Prenatal diagnosis of congenital disorders. In: Creasy RK, Resnick R, Iams JD, et al, editors. Creasy & Resnick's maternal-fetal medicine. 6th edition. Philadelphia: Saunders Elsevier; 2009. p. 222.

2. Tabor A, Vestergaard CH, Lidegaard O. Fetal loss rate after chorionic villus sampling and amniocentesis: an 11-year national registry study. Ultrasound Obstet Gynecol 2009;34:19–24.

3. Nakata N, Wang Y, Bhatt S. Trends in prenatal screening and diagnostic testing among women referred for advanced maternal age. Prenat Diagn 2010;30:198–206.

4. National Institute of Child Health and Development National Registry for Amniocentesis Study Group. Mid-trimester amniocentesis for prenatal diagnosis: safety and accuracy. JAMA 1976;236:1471.

5. Simpson LE, Dallaire L, Miller JR, et al. Prenatal diagnosis of genetic disease in Canada: report of a collaborative study. Can Med Assoc J 1976;15: 739–46.

6. Tabor A, Philip J, Madsen M, et al. Randomized controlled trial of genetic amniocentesis in 4606 low-risk women. Lancet 1986;1:1287–93.

7. Tongsong T, Wanapirak C, Sirivatanapa P, et al. Amniocentesis-related fetal loss: a cohort study. Obstet Gynecol 1998;92:64–7.

8. Pitukkijronnakorn S, Promsonthi P, Panburana P, et al. Fetal loss associated with second trimester amniocentesis. Arch Gynecol Obstet 2010;284(4): 793–7.

9. Towner D, Currier RJ, Lorey FW, et al. Miscarriage risk from amniocentesis performed for abnormal maternal serum screening. Am J Obstet Gynecol 2007;196:608.e1–5.

10. Odibo AO, Gray DL, Dicke JM, et al. Revisiting the fetal loss rate after second-trimester genetic amniocentesis. A single center's 16 year experience. Obstet Gynecol 2008;111:589–95.

11. Kalogiannidis I, Petousis S, Prapa S, et al. Amniocentesis-related adverse outcomes in diamniotic twins: is there a difference compared to singleton pregnancies? Eur J Obstet Gynecol Reprod Biol 2011;155:23–6.

12. Cahill AG, Macones GA, Stamilio DM, et al. Pregnancy loss rate after mid-trimester amniocentesis in twin pregnancies. Am J Obstet Gynecol 2009; 200:257, e1–6.

13. Brumfield CG, Lin S, Conner W, et al. Pregnancy outcome following genetic amniocentesis at 11-14 versus 16-19 weeks' gestation. Obstet Gynecol 1996;88:114–8.

14. Saltvedt S, Almstrom H. Fetal loss rate after second trimester amniocentesis at different gestational age. Acta Obstet Gynecol Scand 1999;78:10–4.

15. The Canadian Early and Mid-Trimester Amniocentesis Trial (CEMAT) Group. Randomized trial to assess safety and fetal outcome of early and mid-trimester amniocentesis. Lancet 1998;351:242.

16. Deprest J, Emonds MP, Richter J, et al. Amniopatch for iatrogenic rupture of the fetal membranes. Prenat Diagn 2011;31:661–6.

17. Cardy AH, Torrance N, Clark D, et al. Amniocentesis in the second trimester and congenital talipes equinovarus in the offspring: a population-based record linkage study in Scotland. Prenat Diagn 2009;29: 613–9.

18. Minna T, Mika G, Tiina L, et al. Risk for placental abruption following amniocentesis and chorionic villus sampling. Prenat Diagn 2011;31:410–2.

19. Centers for Disease Control. Chorionic villus sampling and amniocentesis: recommendations for prenatal counseling. MMWR Recomm Rep 1995; 44(Suppl):1–12.

20. Mujezinovic F, Alfirevic Z. Procedure-related complications of amniocentesis and chorionic callous sampling. A systematic review. Obstet Gynecol 2007;110:687–94.

21. Caughey AB, Hopkins LM, Norton ME. Chorionic villus sampling compared with amniocentesis and the difference in the rate of pregnancy loss. Obstet Gynecol 2006;108:612–6.

22. Odibo AO, Dicke JM, Gray DL, et al. Evaluating the rate and risk factors for fetal loss after chorionic villus sampling. Obstet Gynecol 2008;112:813–9.

23. Jackson LG, Zachary JM, Fowler SE, et al. A randomized comparison of transcervical and transabdominal chorionic-villus sampling. N Engl J Med 1992;327:594–8.

24. Silver RK, MacGregor SN, Muhlbach LH, et al. A comparison of pregnancy loss between transcervical and transabdominal chorionic villus sampling. Obstet Gynecol 1994;83:657–60.

25. Firth HV, Boyd PA, Chamberlain P, et al. Severe limb abnormalities after chorion villus sampling at 56-66 days' gestation. Lancet 1991;337:762–3.

26. Burton BK, Schulz CJ, Burd LI. Limb anomalies associated with chorionic villus sampling. Obstet Gynecol 1992;79:726–30.

27. Froster UG, Jackson L. Limb defects and chorionic villus sampling: results from an international registry 1992-94. Lancet 1996;347:489–94.

28. Kuliev A, Jackson L, Froster U, et al. Chorionic villus sampling safety. Report of World Health Organization/EURO meeting in association with the Seventh

International Conference on Early Prenatal Diagnosis of Genetic Diseases. Tel Aviv, Israel, May 21, 1994. Am J Obstet Gynecol 1996;174:807–11.

29. Goldberg JD, Wohlferd MM. Incidence and outcome of chromosomal mosaicism found at the time of chorionic villus sampling. Am J Obstet Gynecol 1997;176:1349–53.

30. Buscaglia M, Ghisoni L, Bellotti M, et al. Percutaneous umbilical blood sampling: indication changes and procedure loss rate in a nine years' experience. Prenat Diagn 1996;11:106–13.

31. Weiner CP, Okamura K. Diagnostic fetal blood sampling-technique-related losses. Fetal Diagn Ther 1996;11:169–75.

32. Ghidini A, Sepulveda A, Lockwood CJ, et al. Complications of fetal blood sampling. Am J Obstet Gynecol 1993;168:1339–44.

33. Clark TJ, Martin WL, Divakaran TG, et al. Prenatal bladder drainage in the management of fetal lower urinary tract obstruction: a systematic review and meta-analysis. Obstet Gynecol 2003;102: 367–82.

Ultrasound-Guided Transvaginal Interventions in the Pelvis

Gia A. DeAngelis, MD

KEYWORDS

- Pelvis • Transvaginal intervention • Trocar technique • Seldinger technique

KEY POINTS

- Choice of approach to pelvic masses and collections depends on location and need for long-term drainage.
- In an endovaginal approach, the trocar technique is usually easier to perform than the Seldinger technique.
- Placement of a catheter via an endovaginal approach may require modification to the biopsy guide to free the device from the catheter after placement into the collection.
- Effective drainage can be done using multiple aspirations or using a single catheter placement, and choice may depend on the size and viscosity of the fluid collection.
- Assessment of the likelihood of malignancy should be considered before aspiration of an ovarian cyst.

 The author has provided several related videos at http://www.ultrasound.theclinics.com/.

The endovaginal approach using a transvaginal transducer and guide is often the most optimal route to visualize and access central and posterior pelvic lesions. Endovaginal aspiration, biopsy, and catheter placements are very well tolerated, and complications are infrequent.

APPROACHES TO PELVIC MASSES AND COLLECTIONS

Access to pelvic masses and collections can be done percutaneously by a transabdominal (anterior), transgluteal (posterior), or transperineal approach, or by a transvaginal or transrectal endocavitary approach. If accessible, drainage and catheter placement from an anterior percutaneous approach is generally preferred, given patient comfort and physician expertise and the ability to place a larger catheter. Access may be done through the anterior abdominal wall musculature or by traversing the iliacus muscle.

Likewise, a computed tomography (CT)-guided transgluteal approach is also frequently used for similar reasons. This approach is best for pelvic fluid collections posterior to the rectum in the presacral space and ischiorectal fossa and large central pelvic collections. The catheter should be placed medially to avoid the sciatic nerve branches and vessels in the greater sciatic foramen.

Pelvic metastases and collections commonly occur dependently in the rectouterine pouch (the peritoneal recess between the uterus and rectum) and the central pelvis, and are often difficult to access percutaneously given intervening broad ligament, bladder, and bowel. Their proximity to the vaginal fornices makes the transvaginal route an ideal approach.

An endorectal approach has also been used for collections posterior to the rectum. Infection has been infrequent with the use of preprocedure and postprocedure broad-spectrum antibiotics

Department of Radiology, University of Virginia Health System, Box 800170, Charlottesville, VA 22908, USA
E-mail address: GAD9A@Virginia.edu

Ultrasound Clin 7 (2012) 337–345
doi:10.1016/j.cult.2012.03.002

and by effectively aspirating and lavaging the collection.[1,2] In small children unable to tolerate an ultrasound guide transrectally, an alternative is to introduce the catheter with a finger and use sonographic guidance from the anterior pelvis using the full bladder as an acoustic window. A transperineal route is ideal for patients with an abdominoperineal resection.

INDICATIONS FOR TRANSVAGINAL BIOPSY AND ASPIRATION OF SIMPLE COLLECTIONS
Biopsy of Presumed Metastatic Disease

Ovarian, gastrointestinal, and breast malignancies commonly recur as drop metastases to the pelvic floor or ovaries. Small metastases in the central pelvis (**Fig. 1**) may only be accessible by transvaginal biopsy. Because of the usually solid and fixed nature of the metastasis and the short access allowed by the transvaginal approach, transvaginal biopsies are overall the easiest and fastest biopsies to perform. Small recurrences at the vaginal cuff are often poorly resolved with CT but well are visualized with transvaginal ultrasonography, allowing greater confidence in sampling.

Biopsy of Possible Primary Ovarian Neoplasm

Aspiration or biopsy of a potentially malignant cystic ovarian mass is infrequently indicated, given the potential risk of peritoneal seeding. Preliminary consultation with a gynecologic oncologist should be considered. Aspiration of cyst fluid alone often gives false-negative results. If possible, solid components should additionally be sampled to increase positive yield. A partly cystic metastasis may need to be partially drained to allow adequate sampling of solid portions.

INDICATIONS FOR TRANSVAGINAL ASPIRATION OF NONINFECTED FLUID COLLECTIONS
Therapeutic Aspiration of Simple Cysts

Large symptomatic ovarian cysts are usually surgically managed, as they usually recur after simple aspiration.[3,4] However, aspiration may be indicated to reduce risk of torsion or alleviate pain in patients at higher surgical risk, including pregnant patients, or in a patient with one ovary for whom surgical resection can result in infertility or hormonal loss. Instillation of methotrexate[5] or other sclerosants into a cyst after aspiration reduces frequency of recurrence (**Fig. 2**).

A cyst should be determined to be nonneoplastic; the 2009 Society of Radiologists in Ultrasound consensus guideline[6] can be used. If clear, the aspirated fluid is normally not sent for further analysis.

Therapeutic Aspiration of Simple Fluid Collections

Symptomatic relatively simple pelvic fluid collections usually can be completely drained. Simple fluid collections are usually seromas, lymphoceles, peritoneal inclusion cysts, or a hydrosalpinx. Their likely cause and risk of recurrence can be inferred by their appearance on ultrasonography and pertinent clinical history including relation to prior surgery.

Peritoneal inclusion cysts and lymphoceles usually recur after aspiration. In patients at risk for surgery, percutaneous sclerotherapy from a percutaneous or endocavitary approach can be attempted.[7,8]

A postoperative hemorrhage liquefies over time to become a seroma. Aspiration of a seroma is usually complete, and recurrence is unlikely.

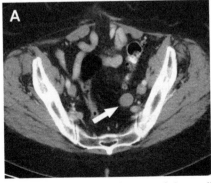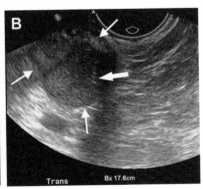

Fig. 1. (*A*) A 60-year-old woman with history of clear cell ovarian cancer. A new 1.8-cm left pelvic lesion (*arrow*) on CT was a suspected first recurrence. (*B*) The lesion (*thin arrows*) was easiest to access via an endovaginal approach. With pressure in the vaginal fornix, the lesion is only 1.3 cm deep to the mucosa of the vaginal fornix. The needle (*large arrow*) tracked close to the expected biopsy path. Both the solid and fluid components were aspirated, yielding cells diagnostic for malignancy.

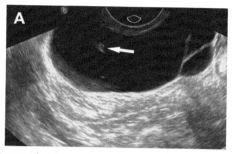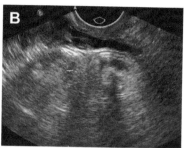

Fig. 2. A patient with a large simple hydrosalpinx (A) had pain related to intermittent torsion. It recurred after a prior aspiration. An 18-gauge needle (*arrow*) was introduced endovaginally and the hydrosalpinx was aspirated completely (B). A sclerosant (180 mg of sodium tetradecyl sulfate in a total volume of 12 mL) admixed with room air was injected into the cyst cavity and the needle withdrawn. No recurrence was seen when followed up a year later.

TRANSVAGINAL DRAINAGE OF INFECTED COLLECTIONS

Indications for drainage include the presence of a large collection not expected to respond to or which has failed antibiotic therapy, a patient with systemic infection, or a patient who has failed a trial of antibiotic therapy. As a general rule, collections under 3 cm are likely to respond to antibiotics alone.

Treatment of Tubo-Ovarian Abscess

Tubo-ovarian abscess (TOA) is usually a polymicrobial infection in women of reproductive age that begins in the fallopian tube from the normal uterine flora and secondarily involves the ovary and, in advanced cases, the adjacent bowel, bladder, and contralateral tube and ovary. Acute TOA is characterized by particulate fluid in a dilated tube with walls thicker than 5 mm and thick, edematous endosalpingeal folds.[9] A chronic TOA usually has thinner walls (<5 mm), less particulate fluid, and more defined walls.

Broad-spectrum antibiotic therapy covering multiple aerobic and anaerobic organisms is the first line of therapy; the regimen may include doxycycline with cefotetan, or clindamycin and gentamycin. Parenteral therapy is usually given for at least 24 hours and is switched to oral therapy after clinical improvement.

Antibiotic therapy fails in approximately 25% of cases, necessitating drainage. Surgical drainage and debridement may compromise fertility and ovarian function, and has a higher risk of complications including bowel perforations.[10]

Ultrasound-guided transvaginal drainage is equally effective as surgical drainage. The transvaginal approach allows the most direct route to a TOA, and allows more precise placement of needles and catheters. Procedure-related complications are rare, and the procedure is well tolerated.

Aspiration alone or catheter placement and drainage are both highly effective in TOA[11] as well as in other infected pelvic collections (**Fig. 3**A).[12]

Treatment of Other Complex Fluid Collections

Infected pelvic collections are also most frequently result from superinfection of pelvic hemorrhage following abdominal and pelvic gynecologic or bowel surgery, and less frequently are due to appendicitis or diverticulitis. Infected hematomas are likely to be very complex, containing both pus and components of undrainable nonliquefied hemorrhage, and usually are more effectively drained over days with a catheter (see **Fig. 3**B).

A periappendiceal or diverticular abscess may completely respond to aspiration or catheter drainage alone. If surgery is eventually required, the initial drainage may allow subsequent surgery to be a 1-step procedure without an interim colostomy. An interloop abscess may not be accessible by any means without traversing the bowel. Aspiration of the collection by traversing a loop of small bowel has been performed with similar therapeutic success.[13]

If a CT scan demonstrates likely continued communication with bowel as in a diverticular abscess or anastomotic leak, a catheter placed in the abscess close to the open communication increases the likelihood that the communication can spontaneously close without surgery. A percutaneous approach should be attempted, given the expected longer time the catheter may need to be in place as the fistula closes.

ASPIRATION VERSUS CATHETER PLACEMENT
Treatment by Aspiration Alone

Advantages are a simple, quick, and less painful procedure, and the ability to treat most women in one session without subsequent catheter management. Disadvantages are the need for repeat

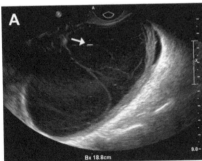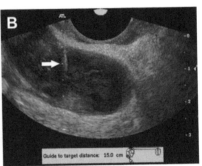

Fig. 3. (A) A patient with a tubo-ovarian abscess responded successfully to antibiotic therapy. The acute inflammation resolved but a dilated hydrosalpinx resulted, and aspiration was requested to relieve pain from intermittent torsion. The fine particulate echoes, thin septations, and decreased thickness of the wall and folds reflect a more chronic process. Complete aspiration yielded 300 mL of clear brown fluid. The cross-hatch (arrow) indicates the length of the needle needed to reach this point. (B) In another patient, a postoperative infected hematoma with complex partially liquefied contents required catheter placement. Aspiration (arrow) yielded purulent bloody fluid. A 10F catheter was subsequently placed using the trocar technique. The hematoma was partially drained initially with the catheter and drainage was near complete over the next 4 days, so the catheter was removed.

aspirations in incompletely drained or recurrent collections. A longer course of antibiotic therapy may be needed given the longer time it takes for the fluid to resolve.

Management by aspiration alone has been highly successful. In one large series of women with TOA, 93% were successfully treated with antibiotics and aspiration alone, although one-third required more than one aspiration.[14] Appropriate selection of patients with a single collection with minimally viscous fluid will increase the likelihood that a single aspiration will completely drain fluid and not need to be repeated.

Purulent fluid can be aspirated though a 16-gauge or 18-gauge needle. Repetitively injecting and aspirating aliquots of sterile saline may effectively remove most of the fluid. Without a catheter, the patient may need to be more closely monitored for reaccumulation of fluid, and repeat aspiration may be necessary.

Treatment Using Catheter Placement

Catheter treatment of an infected collection is also highly successful. Catheter placement should be considered when the collection is large or multiloculated, when there are multiple adjacent collections, or when the collection appears too complex to be drained by aspiration alone. The fluid in multiple or multiloculated collections is likely to drain over time through a catheter as the fluid becomes less viscous with repeated flushes and interim antibiotic therapy.

Catheter placement also has the advantage of being able to more completely empty a complex collection immediately or over days. A single catheter placement is almost always effective.

During the initial placement, manipulation of the wire and catheter and repeated irrigations are more likely to break up very complex collections. The larger holes of a catheter allow complex fluid to be more completely aspirated. Once the catheter is placed, daily repeated flushes also continue to break up complex fluid and lower the viscosity of the fluid.

Transvaginal catheter placement is best accomplished by the trocar method as dilatation and manipulation of dilators over a wire is very difficult transvaginally.

EQUIPMENT
Table

The procedure is performed in the ultrasound suite. A dedicated lithotomy table allows free range of motion of the endovaginal transducer. The transducer handle may need to be dropped lower than the midline coronal plane of the pelvis to visualize lesions at or anterior to the vaginal fornices.

When a dedicated table is unavailable or when the procedure is performed in fluoroscopy, placing a pillow under the buttocks may allow sufficient range of motion of the transducer.

Ultrasonography

The transvaginal transducer should have an attachable guide. Depending on the manufacturer, this may be a single-component or multiple-component system. Most are multiple component where a snap-on disposable guide is attached to a reusable or disposable base. A sterile plastic cover is placed either under or over the guide as appropriate. Most guides allow at least a 16-gauge needle.

Software for the specific transducer should display an on-screen expected needle path.

Needles and Catheters

The needle or catheter should be able to extend beyond the tip of the transducer by at least 2 cm. The minimum length of an aspirating needle or catheter is determined by the length of the biopsy guide plus the distance from the end of the guide to the lesion. Software will indicate the total distance from the end of the guide to the chosen point in the lesion (usually indicated by a cross-hatch on a dotted line on the screen), thus indicating the minimum needle length required (see **Fig. 3**A). Most guides require a length of either 15 cm or 20 cm.

For fine-needle aspiration (FNA), 20-gauge or 22-gauge needles are used. A 22-gauge needle will often provide as much material for cytology as a 20-gauge needle with the advantage of a less bloody specimen, a preference when preparing slides. For therapeutic aspiration, a larger-gauge needle is used. A 20-gauge aspirating needle is often adequate for simple small collections but 18-gauge needles are chosen for large or more complex collections. Core biopsy devices used are usually 16-gauge or 18-gauge.

For catheter placements, 10F or 12F locking pigtail catheters usually suffice in most collections. Most series have used catheters no greater than 10F. A 10F catheter can usually be placed using the preferred single-stick trocar method. For the infrequent collection for which a larger-gauge catheter is needed or the trocar method fails, a Seldinger technique using dilator exchanges may be attempted using both ultrasound and fluoroscopic guidance. For the Seldinger technique, an 18-gauge Chiba needle can accommodate up to a 0.038-in (0.965-mm) guide wire. An extra-stiff guide wire is usually needed given the difficulties using this technique endovaginally.

PREPARATION

Preprocedure consent, sedation, and coagulation screen are similar to those for other procedures, and may additionally include detailing of a possible bladder or bowel injury.

Antibiotics

Series have not reported significant infection rate without the use of antibiotics during aspiration and biopsy of uninfected collections. However, if prophylactic antibiotics are chosen, they are usually given just before the procedure and for 5 days postprocedure. Broad-spectrum antibiotics should cover the expected vaginal flora of gram-positive and gram-negative bacteria. Intravenous gentamycin and clindamycin are common regimens. After the procedure, oral clindamycin for 5 days has good anaerobic coverage. Patients are usually already receiving empiric broad-spectrum antibiotics when drainage is requested.

Sedation

Although a biopsy or aspiration is usually not painful, standard sedation with intravenous midazolam hydrochloride and fentanyl citrate during the procedure helps with anxiety. Catheter placements can be more painful, and are best performed with conscious sedation.

TECHNIQUE: BIOPSY AND ASPIRATION
Bladder

It is best that the bladder be emptied just before the procedure to improve access to lesions. If the patient cannot empty the bladder, a Foley catheter may sometimes be required.

Planning Ultrasonography

A preprocedure scan is performed to ensure the lesion is easily visible and accessible for needle placement. The guide is usually not yet attached to the transducer for patient comfort.

The planned trajectory is examined for intervening bowel or bladder. The bladder is more likely to be in the way and may need to be reemptied. Turning the transducer 180° may also allow a safe trajectory to the lesion, avoiding the bladder.

Sterilization

The perineum is cleaned with 4 × 4 sponges of 10% povidone-iodine or chlorhexidine. Antiseptic-soaked swabs are introduced into the vagina without a speculum, with the expectation that the solution will pool dependently in the vaginal fornices. Alternatively, swabs or 4 × 4 sponges can be introduced into the vagina using forceps or surgical sponge holders with or without a speculum.

Anesthetic

A 10-mL syringe with local anesthetic (2% lidocaine hydrochloride) is attached to a 22-gauge or 20-gauge needle. Care should be taken to push out any air in the needle before anesthetizing, as a small amount of air injected into the soft tissues can create ultrasound artifact, thus decreasing visibility of the lesion.

Biopsy or Aspiration

Use of firm consistent pressure distends the vaginal fornix over the transducer end and helps pin the lesion in place. The planned biopsy trajectory is oriented as perpendicular as possible to the center of the lesion or fluid collection. Firm pressure and a perpendicular orientation will help prevent small mobile solid lesions or ovarian cysts from rolling away from the path of the planned biopsy (**Fig. 4**).

With the transducer held firmly in position, local anesthetic is injected through the guide into the vaginal wall. The needle tip usually can be seen indenting the wall of the vagina.

The needle planned for biopsy or aspiration is then introduced while the transducer is still held firmly in the same position so that it is likely to traverse the desensitized area. It is usually necessary to give a quick forceful jab to introduce the needle into a small or mobile lesion such as a cyst, as either is more likely to roll away from the biopsy trajectory if only slow, gentle pressure is used. If the needle does not immediately penetrate the vaginal wall, the wall may tend away from the needle and degrade the image. It may be necessary to withdraw a little to again obtain a clear image, readjust the trajectory, and give another quick jab.

For an aspiration, the same needle can be used for local anesthetic and then advanced further for aspiration. In this case, a larger gauge (20- or 18-gauge) can be initially chosen for both anesthesia and aspiration.

FNA can be performed using repeated sticks with individual needles or by using a coaxial technique whereby an introducer is first advanced close to or into the lesion and sequential biopsies are done through the introducer. A coaxial approach is generally preferred when access to the lesion is difficult as in a lung biopsy. Use of multiple individual needles is usually preferable in transvaginal biopsies because the lesions are easy to relocate, the thinner needles are better able to penetrate into a mobile lesion, and different areas of the lesion can be sampled.

Specimens

An on-site cytopathologist can determine the adequacy of FNA and help guide allocation of tissue for further studies. A modified Wright stain is used because it allows for quick preparation. In general, the remaining sample can be split between Papanicolaou stains and RPMI medium. Aspirated fluid may be sent for microbiological or chemical analysis. Specific laboratory analysis can help sort out simple collections such as lymphoceles and seromas.

Based on the initial review, the cytopathologist will recommend the need for core-needle biopsy. Cores are often unnecessary in patients with a prior known malignancy or in neoplasms with distinctive cytology, but are useful to visualize the histologic architecture of a lesion. Tissue from core-needle biopsies or RPMI medium can be used for further studies, including immunohistochemical or molecular analysis. Often immunohistochemistry will be the only means to establish a definitive diagnosis in cases with poorly differentiated histology. In addition, immunohistochemistry is used in some treatment protocols, such as for breast cancer.

TECHNIQUE: CATHETER PLACEMENT
Trocar Technique

The trocar technique is generally preferred with endovaginal catheter placements because the stiff introducer is better at stabilizing a catheter than the wire used in the Seldinger technique.

The Seldinger technique is less frequently performed transvaginally because the dilators and catheter are more likely to buckle over the wire given the elasticity of the vaginal mucosa, the inability to apply manual pressure, and the lack

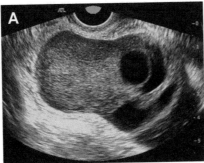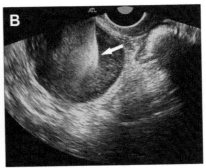

Fig. 4. (*A*) Recurrent leiomyosarcoma in the pelvis. Optimal visualization by ultrasonography revealed the cystic solid nature of this mass. (*B*) The lesion was mobile, and firm pressure was needed to keep the lesion in the biopsy trajectory for subsequent needle placement (*arrow*).

of an incision to aid introduction of the dilators. The wire itself can also easily kink or displace out of the collection during the exchanges.

In the trocar technique, a catheter mounted on a stiff, sharp stylet (trocar) is introduced into the collection in a single step in a similar fashion to a needle biopsy. A guide wire is not used and an incision in the fornix is usually not needed. The procedure can be done entirely under ultrasound guidance without using a speculum for direct visualization. This technique works best with the smaller-size 8F to 10F catheters, but may be successful with 12F catheters.

The same steps are followed as for a biopsy or aspiration, except that modifications to the guide tract may be necessary if the central groove is too small and the cover is not removable.[15] A standard size closed tract is too small to accommodate the large size of a catheter and will prevent it from being freed once placed.

A dedicated peel-away sheath can be used. Alternatively, the sheath that is included with the catheter may be of adequate stiffness to hold the catheter in place and can be modified to become a peel-away sheath (**Fig. 5**). Because the plastic sheath is longer than the catheter, it is shortened to appropriately accommodate the length of the catheter that will extend beyond the guide during placement. As a rule, the catheter should be able to extend at least 5 cm beyond the end of the introducer to take into account the length needed for the tip to coil.

The sheath is slit once lengthwise with a blade and is attached in the groove of the biopsy guide with rubber bands at either end. The end of the sheath should extend close to the tip of the transducer, but may need to be pinched to prevent pain when introduced into the vagina.

Once the transducer is in position in the vagina, the vaginal wall is anesthetized with local anesthetic using a needle passed down the sheath. The same needle can be used to sample the collection. If purulent, the trocar is next introduced through the sheath across the anesthetized tract. The transducer should be held firmly against the vaginal wall to distend the wall and help stabilize the trocar as it is pushed through the vaginal wall and then into the collection.

Once in the collection, the catheter is disengaged from the trocar and the trocar is retracted as adequate catheter coils within the collection. The pigtail is then locked. The transducer is then slowly pulled out of the vagina as the sheath is peeled away to free the catheter as it is being retracted. Other guide attachments for catheters have been described, including an open guide or a guide with a removable cover.

Trocar Technique with a Skin Incision

A skin incision is normally not necessary, as the sharp trocar more easily penetrates the thinner vaginal mucosa than it does the skin. The trocar technique may fail when the elasticity of the vagina is occasionally excessive, as in a young patient, or when a suboptimal angle makes the catheter itself buckle up on the stiff inner stylet as both are being pushed through the vaginal wall. A forniceal incision using a speculum and long-handled blade can help in these occasions. A coronal incision 5 to 10 mm in depth and 3 to 4 mm in width is adequate. The tip of the catheter is introduced into the incision under direct visualization and advanced slightly. Once the tip is within the incision, the transvaginal transducer in inserted and further advancement of the trocar is done under ultrasound guidance.

Seldinger Technique

The Seldinger technique may need to be attempted when a larger catheter is infrequently needed to drain a very complex collection.

In the Seldinger technique, a guide wire is introduced through a needle (usually 18-gauge) and serial dilatations are performed over the wire before catheter placement. The Seldinger is the technique most often used in percutaneous catheter placements, as it allows serial enlargement of a tract so that the catheter easily passes through the tissues over the wire. Pressure is held against the skin during the serial dilatations to prevent kinking of the guide wire and dilators. In addition, the external skin itself is a stable platform for exchanges. However, this technique is very difficult in the mobile vaginal wall where manual pressure cannot be applied. A critical difficulty is lack of an incision; this can be overcome with the following specific modifications.

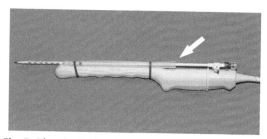

Fig. 5. The plastic sheath is slit lengthwise (*arrow*). The sheath is attached into the groove meant for the manufacturer-specific biopsy guide and attached at either end with rubber bands. A 10-gauge catheter is in locked position and shown within the plastic sheath. The length of the sheath was cut so it can allow at least 5 cm of catheter to extend beyond its end.

An 18-gauge needle is introduced into the collection by ultrasound guidance using the same technique as for a biopsy. The fluid is sampled and a 0.038-in wire placed. A stiffer wire (Amplatz extra stiff, Cook, or Boston Scientific) will ensure a greater likelihood of it remaining in the collection during dilatation.

Subsequent dilatations and catheter placement can be done under fluoroscopic or ultrasound guidance. Fluoroscopy is usually used because the wire is prone to kinking or migrating during serial dilatations and catheter placement, particularly without a vaginal wall incision. If fluoroscopic guidance is planned, iodinated contrast dye (approximately 5 mL) should be injected through the 18-gauge needle before placement of the guide wire.

A forniceal incision can also be made to facilitate passage of the dilators and catheter, similar to that described for the trocar method. The needle is placed into the incision and partially advanced. Further advancement into the collection is done by ultrasound or fluoroscopic guidance. Because of the greater ease in passing serial dilators and a catheter through an incision, ultrasound guidance alone may be possible.

Another modification is use of a Colapinto needle (Cook, Bloomington, IN). A fascial dilator is first mounted onto a Colapinto needle and both are advanced together over the guide wire.[12,16] The Colapinto needle is very stiff, and acts in similar way to a trocar in preventing buckling of the dilator over the more flexible wire. Subsequent catheter placement is then easier, as the tract is more effectively dilated in the absence of an incision.

Irrigation of the Collection

Irrigation of the collection just after catheter placement helps break up debris, and additional fluid may be aspirated. Small 5- to 10-mL aliquots of saline may be repeatedly injected and manually withdrawn to reduce viscosity of the collection and increase drainage. The introduced fluid should not be greater than what was aspirated, to decrease the risk of bacteremia and sepsis from elevated intracavitary pressure.

Thrombolytic Therapy

Adjuvant thrombolytic therapy can be used to further break down fibrin in complex collections in order to facilitate drainage. The risk of bleeding complications is reported to be low in the abdomen and pelvis, given the walled containment of the collection and the short half-life of these agents. The thrombolytic agent and dosage varies among series. For tissue plasminogen activator,

approximately 4 to 6 mg in 25 to 50 mL of saline twice a day for 3 days can be effective. The amount of saline should not be greater than what was removed from the collection.

Catheter Care

Even with the pigtail locked, there is a higher likelihood that a transvaginal catheter can dislodge given the inability to secure the catheter to the vaginal wall close to where it was introduced. The externalized portion of the catheter can instead be attached to the inner thigh using a nonsuture retention adhesive dressing.

Flushing the catheter with 5 to 10 mL of saline 2 to 3 times per day will help ensure that a catheter in a complex collection does not irreversibly clog with debris. Continued antibiotic therapy further expedites resolution of fluid.

Catheter Removal

The catheter may be removed when drainage is small (<10 mL per day) and/or the patient's clinical symptoms and laboratory values normalize. Ultrasonography can be performed to access any residual fluid, but the catheter is often removed without imaging confirmation. Patients tolerate follow-up diagnostic transvaginal ultrasonography even with a catheter in place.

For continued symptoms or continued larger volume or purulent drainage, a CT scan may be needed to access for undrained collections or bowel communication.

COMPLICATIONS

Few major complications have been reported after biopsy, aspiration, or catheter placements. Risk of bleeding is very low. The greatest risk is the introduction of infection.

The trocar technique is theoretically at greater risk of perforating the bowel or bladder, given the pressure needed to traverse the vaginal wall in the absence of a guide wire.

SUMMARY

An endovaginal approach is often the preferred route in aspirating central pelvic collections or biopsy of small lesions. Collections can be managed with aspiration alone. A catheter is considered when the collection is particularly large or complex. The 1-step trocar technique is preferable overall given that it can be performed quickly and entirely under ultrasound guidance, is usually successful, and can be learned rapidly.

SUPPLEMENTARY DATA

Supplementary data related to this article can be found online at doi:10.1016/j.cult.2012.03.002.

REFERENCES

1. Kuligowska E, Keller E, Ferrucci JT. Treatment of pelvic abscesses: value of one-step sonographically guided transrectal needle aspiration and lavage. AJR Am J Roentgenol 1995;164:201–6.

2. Savander BL, Hamper UM, Sheth S, et al. Pelvic masses: aspiration biopsy with transrectal us guidance. Radiology 1990;176:351–3.

3. Duke D, Colville J, Keeling A, et al. Transvaginal aspiration of ovarian cysts: long-term follow-up. Cardiovasc Intervent Radiol 2006;29:401–5.

4. Lipitz S, Seidman DS, Menczer J, et al. Recurrence rate after fluid aspiration from sonographically benign-appearing ovarian cysts. J Reprod Med 1992;37:845–8.

5. Mesogitis S, Daskalakis G, Pilalis A, et al. Management of ovarian cysts with aspiration and methotrexate injection. Radiology 2005;235:668–73.

6. Levine D, Brown DL, Andreotti RF, et al. Management of asymptomatic ovarian and other adnexal cysts imaged at US. Radiology 2010;256:943–54.

7. Lee BC, McGahan JP, Bijan B. Single-step transvaginal aspiration and drainage for suspected pelvic abscesses refractory to antibiotic therapy. J Ultrasound Med 2002;21:731–8.

8. Kim SH, Kim SH, Han H, et al. Image-guided transvaginal drainage of pelvic abscesses and fluid collection using a modified Seldinger technique. Acta Radiol 2008;49:718–23.

9. Timor-Tritsch IE, Lerner JP, Monteagudo A, et al. Transvaginal sonographic markers of tubal inflammatory disease. Ultrasound Obstet Gynecol 1998;12:56–66.

10. McNeeley SG, Hendrix SL, Mazzoni MM, et al. Medically sound, cost-effective treatment for pelvic inflammatory disease and tuboovarian abscess. Am J Obstet Gynecol 1998;178:1272–8.

11. Granberg S, Gjelland K, Ekerhovd E. The management of pelvic abscess. Best Pract Res Clin Obstet Gynaecol 2009;23:667–78.

12. Feld R, Eschelman DJ, Sagerman JE, et al. Treatment of pelvic abscesses and other fluid collections: efficacy of transvaginal sonographically guided aspiration and drainage. AJR Am J Roentgenol 1994;163:1141–5.

13. Maher MM, Gervais DA, Kalra MK, et al. The inaccessible or undrainable abscess: how to drain it. Radiographics 2004;24:717–35.

14. Gjelland K, Ekerhovd E, Granberg S. Transvaginal ultrasound-guided aspiration for treatment of tuboovarian abscess: a study of 302 cases. Am J Obstet Gynecol 2005;193:1323–30.

15. McGahan JP, Wu C. Sonographically guided transvaginal or transrectal pelvic abscess drainage using the trocar method with a new drainage guide attachment. AJR Am J Roentgenol 2008;191:1540–4.

16. Eschelman DJ, Sullivan KL. Use of a Colapinto needle in US-guided transvaginal drainage of pelvic abscesses. Radiology 1993;186:893–4.

Ultrasound-Guided Abdominal and Pelvic Abscess Drainage

Harun Ozer, MD[a],*, Wael E. Saad, MBBCh, FSIR[b]

KEYWORDS

- Ultrasound • Abdominal abscess • Pelvic abscess • Drainage

KEY POINTS

- Ultrasound must be supplemented with fluoroscopy for guidance of catheter deployment if ultrasound depicts only part of an abscess or if more precise catheter positioning is required because of the proximity of adjacent structures. Fluoroscopy is useful to monitor wire manipulations in catheters placed with the Seldinger technique.
- Changes in the character of the drained fluid may be the first indication of a fistula, and further imaging may then be indicated.
- Intrahepatic/parenchymal bile collections (especially after liver transplantation) should be interrogated with contrast and fluoroscopy to assess communication with the biliary tract for both diagnostic and therapeutic purposes.
- In liver transplants, the hepatic artery must be interrogated for hepatic arterial problems, which are common causes for parenchymal infarction, breakdown, and biloma formation.

INTRODUCTION

Abdominal and pelvic abscesses are associated with considerable morbidity among the hospital population.[1] Many cases resolve with antibiotics. However, some are complicated, leading to dissemination of infection with occasional fatal outcome. Antibiotic therapy is the mainstay. However, antibiotic therapy is not always successful because of resistant organisms and/or the presence of large-sized collections.[2] Traditional surgical drainage has been the standard of care in managing these cases. However, surgical drainage has a high operative morbidity and the need for general anesthesia. The availability of minimally invasive image-guided percutaneous drainage has been a major breakthrough, with a lower morbidity and a lesser need for general anesthesia.[2,3] This breakthrough has led to the wider application of percutaneous drainage techniques, with their improvements to safety and efficacy, and has made percutaneous drainage the primary method of managing abscesses. This primary management can be definitive or as a prelude to a more planned and elective subsequent surgery (**Fig. 1**) that has a lower surgical morbidity and mortality.[4]

This article reviews indications and contraindications of percutaneous abscess drainage. In addition, technical considerations are discussed, including the choice of imaging modality for guidance, catheter insertion techniques, methods of catheter fixation and management, techniques for draining abscesses in difficult locations, postdrainage imaging, and complications. Transvaginal drainage of pelvic collections/abscesses is discussed in a separate article by De Angelis and colleagues elsewhere in this issue.

[a] Department of Radiology, University of Virginia Health System, 1215 Lee Street, PO Box 800170, Charlottesville, VA 22908, USA; [b] Division of Vascular Interventional Radiology, Department of Radiology and Imaging Sciences, University of Virginia Health System, Charlottesville, VA, USA
* Corresponding author.
E-mail address: HO4m@Virginia.edu

Ultrasound Clin 7 (2012) 347–362
doi:10.1016/j.cult.2012.03.007
1556-858X/12/$ – see front matter Published by Elsevier Inc.

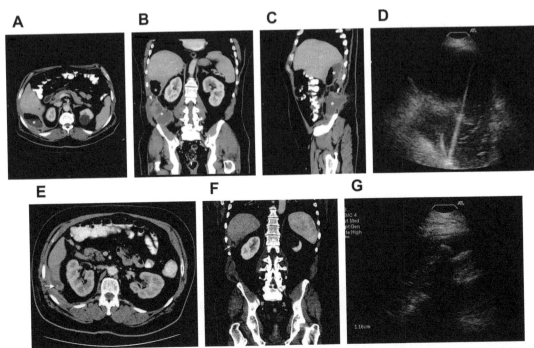

Fig. 1. A 58-year-old man who developed recurrent right upper quadrant abscess extending into the right retroperitoneal space with a remote history of cholecystectomy. (*A*) Axial, (*B*) coronal and (*C*) sagittal contrast-enhanced computed tomography (CT) images of the abdomen show a large, bilobed, peripherally enhancing perihepatic retroperitoneal collection (*white asterisks*) extending from the perihepatic region of the right upper quadrant along the right flank, involving the right paracolic gutter, posterior pararenal space, and lumbar musculature. (*D*) Transabdominal ultrasound image taken during drainage using the Seldinger technique showing catheter looped within the collection. Thick pus was aspirated and the catheter put to bag drainage. (*E*) Axial and (*F*) coronal contrast-enhanced CT images of the abdomen show almost complete resolution of the abscess and a small hyperdense focus (*white arrow*) within the residual abscess cavity at the tip of the liver suspicious for a retained stone. (*G*) Ultrasound shows a 1.3-cm shadowing round focus (between the calipers) within the chronic-appearing inflammatory collection suspicious for a retained gallstone.

INDICATIONS

An abscess is a localized collection of pus in a cavity formed by the disintegration of tissue. Pus is a thick, whitish-yellow fluid that results from the accumulation of white blood cells, liquefied tissue, and cellular debris. Most abscesses are formed by invasion of tissues by bacteria, but some are caused by fungi or protozoa, or even helminths. Other abscesses are sterile (no micro-organism growth on cultures) and are mostly composed of tissue debris. Seventy-five percent of abdominal abscesses are nonvisceral (intraperitoneal or retroperitoneal) and 25% are visceral (hepatic, pancreatic, splenic, renal).[5] There are several factors that predispose to the development of intra-abdominal abscesses. These factors include inflammatory/infectious diseases (cholecystitis, appendicitis, diverticulitis, pancreatitis, Crohn disease), abdominal surgery, abdominal cancer, trauma (blunt or penetrating trauma), and diseases associated with immunologic deficiency.

Although fluid collections have diverse origins, the purposes of percutaneous intervention in all such collections may be classified as 1 or more of the following 3 types: (1) to obtain a fluid sample for diagnosis, (2) to complete drainage of the fluid from an abscess or symptomatic collection, and (3) to treat a recurrent collection by instilling a sclerosing agent.

With respect to diagnosis, aspirated fluid can be sent for laboratory analysis to determine whether it is benign or malignant (for example, cystadenoma vs low-grade cystadenocarcinoma). Microbiologic analysis may reveal an organism as a cause of infection, but, when it does not, a cell count performed on the fluid may help confirm the presence of white blood cells and, thus, infection. A positive result of aspirate culture may provide additional guidance with respect to antibiotic choice, through susceptibility testing of the culture. In some cases, laboratory analysis of a specimen may reveal the cause of the collection; for example, a high creatinine level helps confirm a diagnosis of urinary leak or urinoma

(Fig. 2) and a high bilirubin content helps confirm a diagnosis of biloma or bile leak.

With respect to treatment, abscesses generally require a combination of either percutaneous or surgical drainage and antibiotics for complete cure, because antibiotics usually do not reach sufficient bactericidal concentrations within larger abscess cavities. Very small abscesses, which are usually less than 1 to 3 cm in diameter, frequently resolve with antibiotic therapy alone.[6] In these cases, a period of observation and antibiotic therapy may be appropriate followed by imaging follow-up to ensure resolution of the abscess. To obtain material for culture and susceptibility testing, needle aspiration may be performed (Fig. 3). Infection is not the only indication for drainage. Symptoms such as pain or pressure from a large infected or noninfected fluid collection, or obstruction of adjacent structures (such as bowel or ureter), are also indications for drainage. Patients with abscesses under pressure benefit from the immediate decompression provided by percutaneous drainage. In addition, the percutaneous drainage catheters may also be used as conduits for infusing a sclerosing agent (discussed later) into a recurrent noninfected collection or for

the administration of tissue perfusion activator (tPA) to help drain collections that are recalcitrant to simple percutaneous drain placement (discussed later).[7]

CONTRAINDICATIONS

Contraindications for percutaneous treatment are few. The main ones are uncorrectable coagulopathy, lack of safe percutaneous access, and inability of the patient to cooperate with catheter management after placement (eg, patient removing catheter after catheter placement). For practical purposes, the absence of a safe percutaneous path is the only factor that prohibits percutaneous abscess drainage, because, in most instances, coagulopathy can be corrected to allow drainage. The presence of bowel overlying the abscess may prevent percutaneous abscess drainage (Fig. 4). Abscesses located near or between bowel loops are not amenable to percutaneous catheter drainage and may require surgery if the patient experiences symptoms of peritonitis. However, in the absence of acute peritonitis, needle aspiration of an interloop abscess can be performed to obtain material for culture.

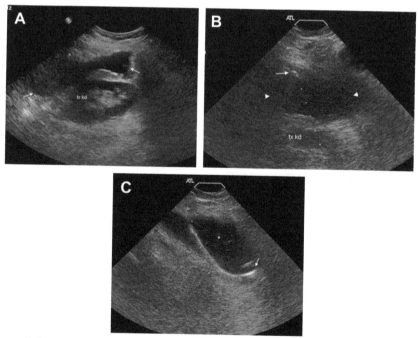

Fig. 2. (A) Gray-scale longitudinal transabdominal ultrasound image showing an elongated loculated collection (between the *white arrows*) anterior to the transplant kidney. (B) Transabdominal ultrasound image taken during a drainage using the Seldinger technique in a patient with a loculated collection in close proximity to a pelvic transplant kidney. The needle (*white arrow*) can be seen correctly placed within the collection (between the catheter looped *white arrow*). (C) Subsequent view showing catheter looped within the collection (*white asterisk*). Clear fluid was aspirated and the catheter left on free drainage. Samples were sent to the laboratory for analysis including creatinine.

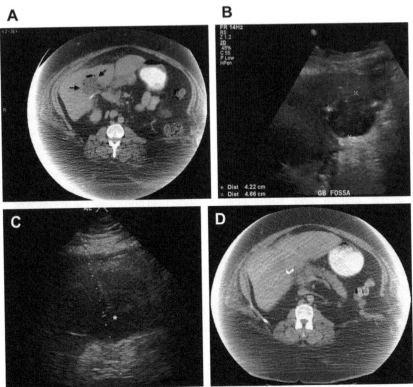

Fig. 3. Images in a 46-year-old woman with a right upper quadrant abscess that occurred after laparoscopic cholecystectomy. (*A*) Axial contrast-enhanced CT and (*B*) transverse ultrasound image shows small abscess (*black arrows* and between the calipers respectively) in the gallbladder fossa. (*C*) Transabdominal ultrasound image taken during aspiration of the abscess (*white asterisk*) using an 18-gauge Chiba needle. The needle can be seen correctly placed within the collection. A total of 40 mL of purulent fluid was aspirated. (*D*) Follow-up contrast-enhanced CT image showing resolution of the abscess in the gallbladder fossa.

Transgression of the small bowel with a fine (22-gauge) needle is generally safe. However, transgression of the colon should be avoided, because the colonic flora will contaminate the specimen

![CT scan figure 4]

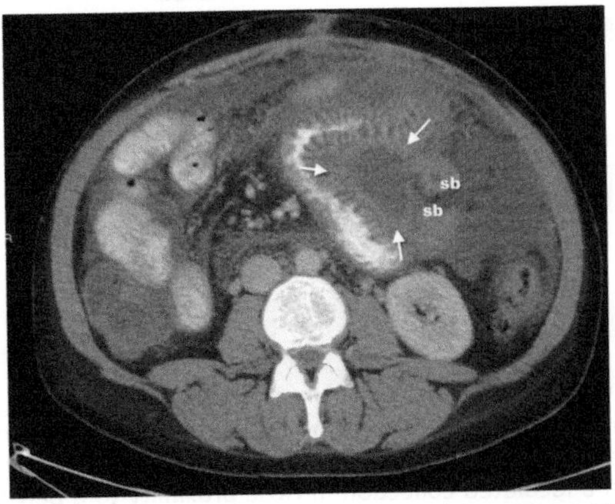

Fig. 4. CT scan obtained in a 32-year-old woman with Crohn disease reveals an interloop abscess (between the *white arrows*) that is inaccessible with percutaneous catheter placement because of multiple bowel loops (sb).

and may cause infection in the fluid collection. Some 18-gauge needles come with blunt stylets, which are used to push bowel away and/or skim past the bowel without catching its walls and injuring the bowel.

IMAGE-GUIDANCE MODALITY

An appropriate choice of imaging modality for guidance is a vital first step because it provides information regarding feasibility, appropriate technique, and associated risks for the purposes of informed consent and procedural planning.[8] The choice depends on physician preference and comfort as well as anatomic factors such as the size of the collection and its location in relation to the surrounding structures. The most straightforward imaging guidance modality for abscess drainage is ultrasonography.[8] Ultrasound allows real-time observation of the abscess, needle placement, and catheter placement, without exposure of the patient to ionizing radiation. In large and readily accessible abscesses, deployment of the catheter by using the trocar technique with real-time ultrasound guidance is the simplest and fastest way to achieve percutaneous drainage. However, if ultrasound depicts only part of an abscess or if more precise catheter positioning is required because of the proximity of adjacent structures, ultrasound must be supplemented with fluoroscopy for guidance of catheter deployment. Fluoroscopy is used to monitor wire manipulations in catheters placed with the Seldinger technique. Limitations of ultrasound include its inability to depict the extent of an abscess in a deep location such as the pelvis. In addition, an abscess that is partially obscured by bowel air can be difficult to localize, and an abscess that contains air may be difficult to see or impossible to differentiate from bowel at ultrasound.

Computed tomography (CT) is the preferred modality to identify the extent of abscesses and to plan the route of access because distinction of the fluid collection from the adjacent normal structures can be enhanced by the administration of oral and intravenous contrast agents. As a result, CT is also advantageous for guiding drainage, particularly in cases in which collections are small and deep, in close proximity to vital structures, and located in regions that are difficult to access (eg, the transgluteal route for pelvic drainage). In addition, CT fluoroscopy assures increased accuracy and decreased procedure time. The major disadvantages of CT guidance are that it is not in real time and that it has a radiation dose. The latter is a particular concern in the pediatric population. Therefore, whenever technically feasible, ultrasound is the primary guidance modality in the pediatric population.

PATIENT PREPARATION

Patient preparation requires evaluation and normalization of coagulation status, administration of periprocedural, culture-specific, or broad-spectrum antibiotics, and evaluation of the patient for tolerance of conscious sedation. Conscious sedation is critical to reduce patient pain and anxiety, increase technical ease and comfort, and thereby decrease the risk of complications. General anesthesia or anesthesiologist-administered sedation may be required in complicated patients with high comorbidities. For some patients, the procedure may be performed with only local anesthetic because the risk of sedation or anesthesia may be greater than the risk of the procedure, which may be the case for patients with the combination of tenuous cardiopulmonary status and a large, superficial fluid collection.

PROCEDURE

Because of the risks of complications such as sepsis, bleeding, and oversedation, abscess drainage should be performed during active monitoring of heart rate, blood pressure, and oxygen saturation. Regardless of the imaging modality used for guidance, there are 2 methods for placement of a catheter into an abscess. Each method has its pros and cons. Operator preferences play a large part in the choice of technique. These techniques are the 1-step trocar technique and the transitional guidewire-based Seldinger technique.[8]

Trocar Technique

This technique involves a catheter mounted on a sharp trocar (nonhypodermic needle) and inserted into the abscess. The accurate placement of the guiding needle is of the utmost importance to ensure the safety of this technique and the accurate positioning and deployment of the drainage catheter, because the drainage catheter is committed as it is placed with the needle as 1 unit (compare with the Seldinger technique, as discussed later). The catheter, mounted on the trocar needle, is then advanced as 1 unit to a premeasured depth. Advantages of this technique include the ability to rapidly deploy (1 step) the drainage catheter, which is essential if the temporal window for sedation is nearing its end. Disadvantages include the difficulty of repositioning a catheter that has been deployed suboptimally on the first pass. Another disadvantage is that small-caliber drainage catheters (<12F) are usually best deployed using this technique and not large-caliber drainage catheters (12F or greater). Furthermore, the fluid collection (abscess) has to be mature with a defined structure and well-formed wall (reactive fibrotic tissue enclosure). If the collection does not have a well-formed wall/weak wall, inappropriate (usually through-and-through) drainage-catheter deployment will occur.

Seldinger Technique

The Seldinger technique involves the insertion of a hollow needle into the abscess cavity and the placement of a guidewire through the needle to create a percutaneous path for a drainage catheter. After the guidewire is inserted, the needle is withdrawn and exchanged for the drainage catheter, which is placed over the wire and inserted into the abscess. The percutaneous deployment of 8F to 14F catheters usually requires the use of 0.89-mm (0.035 in) or 0.97-mm (0.038 in) wires. The needle puncture can be performed with a needle system that accommodates these wires (generally, 18-gauge angiographic needles or 19-gauge needles sheathed in 5F catheters) or with a fine (21-gauge or 22-gauge) needle that accommodates a 0.46-mm (0.18 in) wire. In the latter case, a dilator-and-sheath system is used either to upsize/exchange the 0.46-mm wire for a 0.89-mm or 0.97-mm wire or to insert a 0.89-mm or 0.97-mm working guidewire. Unlike the trocar technique, multiple attempts can be made before committing to the final drainage-catheter placement. Moreover, the Seldinger technique allows the ability to direct the wire to the location desired for catheter deployment. Precise positioning is especially necessary in large abscesses, such as those that occur in the subphrenic region, and in locations in which access is tightly restricted. Disadvantages of the Seldinger technique include the difficulty of working with wires in confined spaces, and the multiple steps involved in dilation. In addition, when dilators and wires are used with ultrasound or CT guidance, any buckling or kinking of the wire can be problematic. If there is a significant kink in the guidewire, it usually needs to be exchanged for a new guidewire. Leakage from small fluid collections around the wire during needle removal and dilations may substantially reduce operating space in the abscess and make catheter placement more difficult.

Catheter Fixation and Postprocedure Care

Most radiologists use 2 means of catheter fixation: an internal fixation mechanism and an external fixation device. For internal retention, most radiologists use locking pigtail catheters. A string that courses through the catheter is fixed in place near the hub of the drainage catheter; this pigtail reduces the risk of inadvertent catheter dislodgement/discontinuation. The string is made in such a way that it will break under excessive tension or pressure, thus ensuring that the catheter will not rupture inside the patient. Other specially designed external fixation devices have been developed to obviate suturing of the catheter to the patient's skin. Drainage catheters may be taped or sewn to a device that adheres to skin. This method avoids the skin irritation caused by sutures, as well as the need for suture removal.

The abscess cavity is preferably decompressed at the time of drainage with direct suction by using a syringe attached to the catheter. Some operators use a method analogous to surgical lavage and irrigate the abscess cavity with aliquots of 10 to 15 mL of 0.9% saline to encourage further drainage of thick debris.[8] However, irrigation of the abscess must be performed with a lesser volume of fluid than that previously drained from the abscess, to avoid an increase in intracavitary pressure with resultant bacteremia and sepsis. The ability to drain all or most of the fluid collection at the time of initial drainage-catheter placement depends on the viscosity of the fluid within the collection and the degree of necrotic/partly liquefied tissue component within the collection. A simple noninfected fluid collection (lymphocele, for example) can be aspirated completely at the time of initial catheter placement. In contrast, a partly liquefied complex collection (eg, organized hematoma or a pancreatic pseudocyst) requires larger drainage catheters (discussed later) and require longer periods of drainage.[8]

After the catheter is secured in place in the decompressed abscess, the catheter should be flushed every 8 to 12 hours with 5 to 10 mL of saline solution to clear the tube of any adherent plugs, encrustations, or debris that might cause drainage-catheter blockage. The catheter position should be assessed to ensure that the catheter is not withdrawing from the abscess, and the access site and dressing should be carefully examined. Difficulty in flushing a catheter may indicate a blockage.[8] If the abscess is incompletely drained, a clogged catheter will have to be exchanged for a new catheter. Frequent drainage-catheter blockage caused by debris usually requires upsizing of the drainage catheter. Changes in the character of the drained fluid may be the first indication of a fistula, and further imaging may then be indicated. A more pathognomonic sign of a fistula (usually between the collection and the gastrointestinal tract) is continuous drainage output that does not decrease over time and is in excess of the total fluid volume expected to be drained from the collection.[8] The expected volume of a fluid collection can be estimated by multiplying the maximum axial dimension of the collection by 0.52 ($x \times y \times 0.52$ = fluid volume in milliliters). If a fistula is suspected and no sepsis is present, an abscessogram may be obtained via catheter for signs of communication with structures such as the bowel, pancreatic and biliary ducts, or genitourinary system. In the presence of sepsis, this examination is deferred so as not to exacerbate sepsis. Disease processes that commonly have fistula formation with the gastrointestinal tract include pancreatitis (pancreatic pseudocysts), Crohn disease, postoperative bowel abscesses, and colonic diverticulitis.

CONSIDERATIONS FOR SPECIFIC ABSCESS SITES

With a clear percutaneous pathway to the abscess and clear depiction of the abscess by ultrasound, placement of a drainage catheter is straightforward (**Fig. 5**). However, abscesses in some locations may pose special challenges.

Abscesses Located in the Pelvis

It may be difficult to access fluid collections deep in the pelvis, because of anterior bowel, bladder, and uterus; lateral bones and blood vessels; and posterior bones. In such abscess locations, percutaneous access with routine anterior or lateral approaches is often impossible. If an abscess is close to the rectum or vagina, a transrectal or transvaginal approach may be used, respectively. A dedicated article in this issue addresses transvaginal drainage. Dedicated endoluminal ultrasound transducers equipped with specialized hardware may be used with this approach to guide the needle or trocar-catheter into the appropriate position. Some patients may not tolerate insertion of the ultrasound transducer. In such patients, transrectal drainage can still be performed with ultrasound guidance and/or fluoroscopic guidance by using an anterior approach, a routine surface transducer, and bladder distention to create an acoustic window. The operator positions the catheter while observing the real-time ultrasound images. Either the trocar or the Seldinger technique may be used. When considering use of the transrectal approach, which is not sterile, the interventionalist should assess the patient's overall clinical condition to determine whether infection is likely to be present in the fluid collection; the goal is to avoid inducing infection in a sterile fluid collection. Although transrectal catheters may seem awkward at first, they are well tolerated by most patients and permit them to ambulate and use the bathroom as normal. Technical details of transrectal ultrasound-guided procedures are similar to those of transvaginal procedures (see article elsewhere in this issue).

The transgluteal approach through the greater sciatic foramen is an alternative that can be used for deep pelvic abscesses.[6,9] Initially described by Butch and colleagues,[9] the transgluteal approach requires CT or fluoroscopic guidance and patient positioning in either the prone or the decubitus position. The choice of transrectal versus transgluteal access to a deep pelvic abscess is often determined by operator preference. Although the transgluteal approach to posterior pelvic collections is popular in many, but not all, practices, operators must be aware that it is a more painful procedure requiring more sedation.

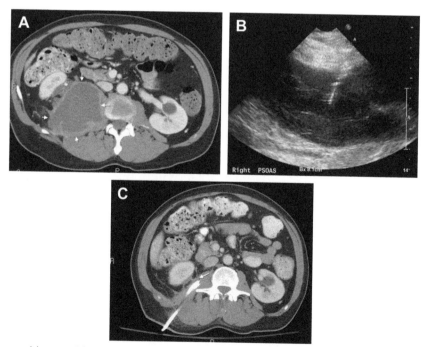

Fig. 5. A 53-year-old man with a recent history of lumbar surgery. (*A*) Contrast-enhanced axial CT image shows a large rim-enhancing low-density lesion consistent with an abscess (between the *white arrows*) in the right psoas muscle extending into the right perirenal space (*white asterisk*). (*B*) Transabdominal ultrasound image taken during abscess drainage; the needle can be seen correctly placed within the collection. (*C*) Follow-up contrast-enhanced axial CT obtained showing complete resolution of the abscess in the right psoas muscle and perirenal space with no residual collection around the pigtail catheter (*white arrow*).

In addition, patients must be informed that it is more likely to be painful after the procedure in 10% to 20% of cases.[9] However, the transgluteal approach has the advantage of allowing percutaneous access to abscesses located farther cephalad where transrectal drainages become difficult, if not impossible, from a safety standpoint. In addition, use of the transgluteal approach is strongly favored in abscesses in which infection is uncertain, because this approach allows drainage while using strict sterile technique.[9]

Abscesses Located in the Subphrenic Area

Subphrenic abscesses may develop after surgery or trauma (**Fig. 6**). For example, a left subphrenic abscess may occur after splenectomy, and a right subphrenic abscess may be related to liver trauma or liver transplantation surgery. In the absence of blunt trauma and history of splenectomy, the most common type of collection in the left subphrenic space is a biloma. When possible, the abscess is drained with a subcostal approach. If there is no possible subcostal percutaneous path to an abscess, intercostal (usually posterior) access may be necessary.[10] The safest intercostal access is the most caudal and anterior approach possible, because the anterior pleural reflection is farther cephalad than the posterior reflection. Most patients who undergo intercostal subphrenic abscess drainage do not develop pleural complications, but all patients should be carefully monitored for such occurrences.[10,11] Subphrenic abscess drainage should ideally be performed by using ultrasound guidance to position a needle in the most caudal aspect of the fluid collection, with the needle tip pointed cephalad to allow the subsequently placed wire to migrate cephalad beneath the diaphragm. The catheter then should be deployed with its tip just below the diaphragm (**Fig. 7**).

Abscesses Located in the Lesser Sac and Peripancreatic Area

The lesser sac region may be difficult to access with an anterior approach because of the stomach, with a lateral approach because of the liver and spleen, and with a posterior approach because of bone and kidneys. The major consideration in choosing imaging modalities and access routes to facilitate percutaneous procedures for lesser sac, pancreatic, or peripancreatic collections is to avoid crossing small or large bowel or major mesenteric, peripancreatic, or retroperitoneal vessels.[12] In small children, thin women, or

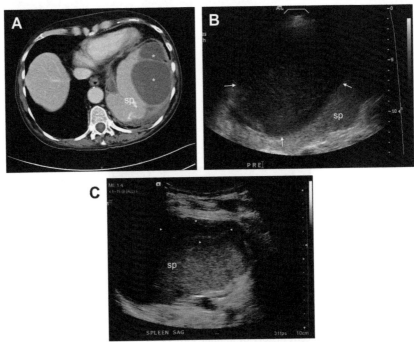

Fig. 6. (*A*) Contrast-enhanced axial CT image of the upper abdomen shows a bilobed subphrenic collection (*white asterisks*) secondary to blunt trauma. (*B*) Transverse gray-scale ultrasound image of spleen (sp) shows a large subphrenic collection (between the *arrows*) compressing the normal splenic parenchyma. (*C*) Follow-up gray-scale ultrasound image of spleen after ultrasound-guided drainage shows minimal residual collection (between the *arrow heads*) and normal uncompressed splenic parenchyma (sp).

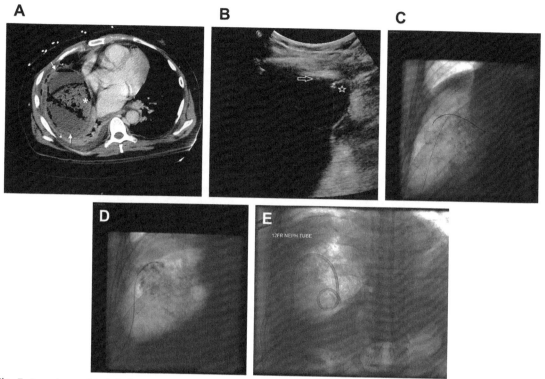

Fig. 7. Imaging-guided drainage of a large subdiaphragmatic abscess with use of the Seldinger technique in a 64-year-old patient status post liver transplant. (*A*) Axial CT image shows a large abscess (between the *white arrows*) and localized hepatic necrosis (*white asterisk*). (*B*) Longitudinal gray-scale ultrasound image of right upper quadrant shows a 21-gauge needle tip (*hollow white arrow*) being inserted into the peritoneal space overlying the right lobe of the liver. Small pockets of air (*white star*) are also seen in inferior aspect of the perihepatic space. (*C*) Fluoroscopic spot film image showing 0.46-mm wire positioned into the subdiaphragmatic collection through a 21-gauge needle. (*D*) Fluoroscopic image with a transitional sheath system in place, which is used to direct a working wire into the largest and farthest cephalic part of the abscess. The position was confirmed with injection of a small amount of contrast. (*E*) On serial dilatation to 12F, a 12F locking pigtail catheter was deployed over the 0.89-mm working wire.

cachectic elderly patients, a paucity of abdominal fat may further limit access. In patients with more abdominal fat, anterior approaches often are used, but other possible approaches include a posterior approach (lateral or medial to the kidneys), transhepatic approach, or transgastric approach. A transhepatic route may be used that transgresses the periphery of the liver (**Fig. 8**). However, a more central transgression of the liver should be avoided because of the large vessels and bile ducts.[13] The liver may also be used as a acoustic window while draining transhepatically. Filling the stomach with sterile water may also allow the stomach to be used as an acoustic window for an ultrasound-guided transgastric approach. Moreover, filling of the stomach may push large and/or small bowel away from the needle access window to the peripancreatic fluid collection.

Despite the advantages of ultrasound guidance, CT guidance is commonly used by many practices

for percutaneous drainage of abscesses in this region, because of the depth of the location and its proximity to vital structures. Because of its vascularity, the spleen is also not generally crossed to reach another target. Likewise, the normal pancreas is not typically transgressed, because of the risk of pancreatitis.

POSTDRAINAGE IMAGING AND DRAINAGE-CATHETER MANAGEMENT
Basic Drainage-Catheter Management and Imaging Follow-up

Many patients need no further imaging after percutaneous abscess drainage of small, simple collections if the clinical course improves and catheter output declines to less than 10 to 20 mL daily. However, persistent fever, pain, or leukocytosis, and/or lack of drainage after percutaneous abscess drainage suggests that further imaging may be needed. CT is most commonly used to

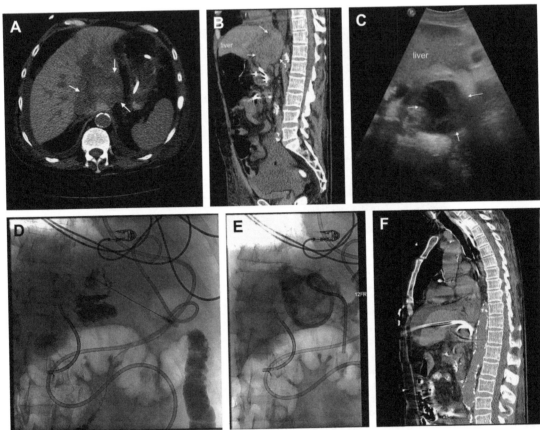

Fig. 8. Transhepatic pancreatic pseudocyst drainage in an 62-year-old man who was deemed unfit for surgery. (*A*) Axial and (*B*) sagittal nonenhanced CT scans show a retroperitoneal heterogeneous collection (between the *white arrows*) secondary to chronic pancreatitis. (*C*) Transverse gray-scale ultrasound shows the pancreatic pseudocyst (between the *white arrows*) using the liver as an acoustic window. (*D*) A 21-gauge needle inserted into the pseudocyst under ultrasound guidance (not shown). Fluoroscopic image with contrast in the pseudocyst confirms the position of the needle and no communication is identifiable with the biliary system. (*E*) Fluoroscopic image with a 12F pigtail catheter is correctly placed within the pseudocyst. Also noted are cystgastrostomy tube, biliary stent, and enteric tube. (*F*) Postprocedure CT scan shows satisfactory catheter position with reduction in pseudocyst size. This approach was used to access a component of the collection located between the liver and the retroperitoneum superior to the pancreas.

monitor the adequacy of drainage, as well as the development of new abscesses. If CT images show that the abscess is completely drained, a decision to remove the catheter may be made, depending on the presence or absence of continued drainage. If there is persistent drainage despite the obliteration of the collection by CT, then a fistula should be suspected and a fluoroscopic contrast study of the drainage catheter is warranted. This contrast fluoroscopic study is termed tube check, tubogram, fistulogram, sinogram, and abscess-check, to name a few.

If CT images show incomplete resolution of the abscess in spite of optimal catheter positioning, then catheter patency should be reassessed with a 5-mL to 10-mL saline flush. If the catheter is patent and well positioned but the abscess persists, the catheter should be exchanged for a larger catheter. Locking pigtail catheters as large as 14 to 16 F are available. In general, the smallest catheter that should be placed initially is 8 or 10 F in adults (6 F in infants), because pus is viscous and will not drain effectively otherwise. If the CT images show that the drainage catheter is no longer in the collection (inadvertent dislodgement or drainage of a locule with residual adjacent collections), a drain repositioning under fluoroscopy and/or an additional de novo percutaneous drain placement is required.

Fistula Imaging and Management

The index of suspicion for fistula should always be high when treating pancreatic abscesses and/or abscesses associated with enteric disorders. The presence of a fistula may be indicated by the underlying disease process or the character of the drained fluid. Conditions such as Crohn disease or pancreatic duct injuries (traumatic and/or pancreatitis-related pancreatic pseudocysts included), which may occur after surgery in the left upper abdominal quadrant, are likely to be associated with fistulas. In addition, the presence of a fistula may be signaled by a change in the appearance of the drained fluid. In the initial period of drainage, most abscesses yield purulent fluid. However, after 2 or 3 days, most of the pus will have drained, and, if a fistula is present, the fluid that follows it will have entered the abscess cavity via the fistula. The drainage volume may increase at this point, and the appearance and viscosity of the fluid will change as a result of its different origin. Fistulas can arise in the gastrointestinal tract, the genitourinary tract, the biliary system, or the pancreatic duct. When a fistula is suspected, a sinogram may be useful for diagnosis and localization. If the suspected fistula is in the bowel, CT may be performed with oral contrast material to confirm the diagnosis. Prolonged drainage may allow a fistula to close, but, in some cases, surgery may be necessary. For prolonged drainage, the drainage catheter needs to be downsized to a minimum over time. Downsizing not only concerns the caliber of the drain (<6 F) but also the placing of straight drains and not the traditional pigtail catheters that preserve a cavity around the pigtail end of the drainage catheter. Adjunctive fibrin seals can be used, although, in the authors' opinion, their effectiveness for fistula healing is questionable. It is imperative to understand that fistula healing relies on numerous factors including many that are not related to imaging/radiology. Factors that hinder fistula healing include, but are not limited to, debilitating diseases, malnutrition, steroid use, and distal bowel or pancreatic duct obstruction. Numerous consults with surgery, nutrition, and stoma/wound care medical providers are therefore required.

In many situations, adjunctive procedures short of open surgery may facilitate fistula healing. For example, in patients with infected bilomas from trauma or iatrogenic causes, sphincterotomy with or without endoscopic biliary stent placement may be performed to facilitate internal drainage of bile and minimize bile leakage into the abscess cavity. Endoscopically placed pancreatic stents help with pancreatic pseudocysts with associated distal pancreatic strictures. Likewise, in patients with urinomas formed by posttraumatic urine leaks, a ureteral stent or a percutaneous nephrostomy catheter may be placed to divert flow away from the urinoma and facilitate closure of the fistula. In patients with a high-output enteral fistula, prolonged parenteral nutrition and exclusion of oral nutrition may be necessary. Abscess recurrence after successful drainage is rare; it is found in less than 5% of patients.[6] In some patients, repeated percutaneous drainage may be successful, but other patients may eventually require surgery.

In rare cases, drainage failure may result from misdiagnosis. Many conditions might cause transient leukocytosis and fever, symptoms that could lead to the misinterpretation of CT findings as abscesses. However, minimal fluid drainage and little change in the appearance of the lesion on images should prompt consideration of other diagnoses, such as low-density tumors. Tumors may also become infected. In these abscesses, the catheters may have to remain in place indefinitely unless the underlying tumor resolves. Patients and referring physicians must be counseled that these drains may remain indefinitely, which is a major source of morbidity to the patient. However, in the setting of superadded infection with systemic infectious dissemination (bacteremia and/or sepsis) operators may, reluctantly, drain infected tumors.

Thrombolytic Assisted Drainage

Adjuvant thrombolytic therapy may be used to break down fibrin/fibrous synechia causing loculations within collections to facilitate drainage.[7] Traditionally, streptokinase in a dose of 120,000 units and, more recently, tissue plasminogen activator (tPA) in a dose of 2 to 10 mg may be administered in normal saline solution. Although there is little reported experience with intracavitary tissue plasminogen activator, abundant anecdotal evidence that accumulated when urokinase was commercially unavailable, from 1998 to 2002, supports its use. Doses of tissue plasminogen activator have not yet been standardized and vary among institutions. The volume of normal saline used may be as much as 50 mL, but it must be adjusted according to the size of the abscess and the volume of fluid drained. The volume instilled should be less than the volume of abscess contents already removed, so as not to place the abscess contents under excessive pressure and risk of sepsis. The thrombolytic agent is left dwelled (drainage catheter clamped) inside the abscess for 20 to 45 minutes and is then allowed to drain. Treatment twice daily for 1 to 3 days is generally effective. CT after a 3-day course may be used to evaluate the effectiveness of thrombolytic therapy and to guide further management. Fibrinolytics should be used with caution (including contrast-enhanced CT investigation) in collections that may be associated with pseudoaneurysms. These clinical scenarios with high risk for pseudoaneurysms include postoperative abscesses for which the surgery involves vascular anastomoses and pancreatic pseudocysts, particularly in the setting of active pancreatitis and in the setting of hemorrhagic pancreatitis.

Sclerosis of Recurrent Sterile Collections

Some collections such as hepatic and renal cysts, lymphoceles, and inclusion cysts may require sclerosis because of recurrence or persistence despite long-term drainage.

Lymphoceles following pelvic surgery are the classic example of collections that tend to recur and may take a long time to drain completely because of persistent leakage from small lymphatics. Many different agents are used, including tetracycline, absolute ethanol (97%–99%), bleomycin, doxycycline, and betadine. It is important to delineate the cavity by injecting contrast through the catheter before starting sclerosis to ensure that there is no communication to bowel, ureter, or other organs (**Fig. 9**).

The collection should be aspirated maximally to rid the collection of its native fluid, to maximize the contact of the subsequent sclerosant instillment with the walls of the collection to reduce the recurrence of fluid accumulation. Less caustic sclerosing agents (tetracycline, bleomycin, doxycycline, and betadine) are instilled to a total of 75% to 90% of the estimated volume of the cavity. More caustic agents (97%–99% ethanol) are instilled to a total of one-third to one-half of the estimated volume of the cavity. The sclerosing agents are left to dwell in the cavity for 45 to

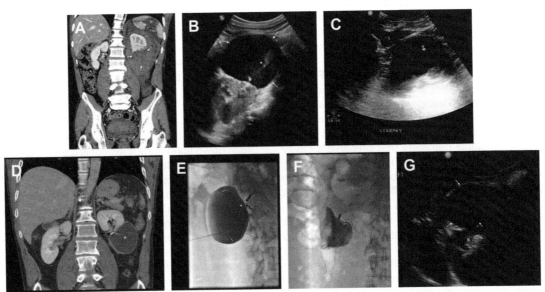

Fig. 9. A 35-year-old man involved in a high-speed motor vehicle crash. (*A*) Contrast-enhanced coronal CT abdomen shows shattered lower pole of the left kidney (lk) (between the *white arrows*) and large hemorrhage (*white asterisks*) in the left retroperitoneal space. (*B*) Follow-up sagittal ultrasound image obtained 3 weeks later shows a well-defined, thin-walled 6.5-cm fluid collection (between the *white arrows*) related to the area of greatest renal injury. Debris (*white asterisk*) is seen layering within the fluid collection. (*C*) An 18-gauge needle tip is being inserted into the posttraumatic cyst within the mid and lower pole of the left kidney, through which 70 mL of straw-colored fluid were aspirated. (*D*) Follow-up contrast-enhanced coronal CT image shows almost the same sized fluid density collection (*white asterisk*) within the mid and lower pole of the kidney, consistent with recurrence of the posttraumatic cyst. (*E*) Second session of cyst aspiration in combination with sclerosis at this time. Fluoroscopic image after 50 mL of clear yellow fluid were withdrawn and 20 mL of contrast (*white asterisk*) were injected into the fluid collection. Double contrast evaluation with air (*white arrows*) showed no communication of the lesion with the collecting system or with the vascular structures of the kidney. (*F*) Fluoroscopic image after 20 mL of dehydrated alcohol was injected and allowed to dwell for 30 minutes. Twenty-two milliliters of fluid and alcohol were withdrawn. Note that the walls of the cyst are collapsed. Coils are also noted, related to prior embolization of branches of the renal artery. (*G*) Follow-up sagittal gray-scale ultrasound in 3 weeks shows significant interval decrease in size of the posttraumatic cyst (between the *white arrows*), which now measures 3.2 cm in the left kidney (lk).

60 minutes, during which the patient turns every 15 minutes into supine, prone, and both decubitus positions. The sclerosing agent is then reaspirated as much as possible. If the collection is small (<5–10 cm), a single session may be sufficient. If the collection is large (>10 cm), sclerosis is repeated for 3 days.

ORGAN-SPECIFIC ABSCESSES AND THEIR CAUSES
Liver Abscesses

Pyogenic liver abscesses are a common indication for percutaneous abscess drainage in the United States. A particularly challenging liver abscess is one that is located cephalad, near the dome of the diaphragm. The optimal guidance modality in these circumstances may be combined ultrasound and fluoroscopy to best achieve the appropriate angulation. CT with an angled gantry can also be used to access these collections. Typical causes for pyogenic liver abscesses include extension of gallbladder and gallstone disease, biliary obstruction (**Fig. 10**), prior trauma or surgery, and seeding from sepsis (eg, appendicitis, diverticulitis).

Although amebic abscesses are preferably treated with antibiotics such as metronidazole, certain situations prompt percutaneous drainage,[14–16] including poor response to antibiotic therapy, uncertainty as to the diagnosis, imminent or even actual leakage or rupture, diameter larger than 6 to 8 cm,[15,17] and left lobe abscesses that have a tendency to rupture into the thorax. Furthermore, pyogenic superinfection of an amebic hepatic abscess can occur, which warrants drainage.[15] Amebic abscesses are usually unilocular and can be drained with ultrasound guidance alone.[18] Catheters need not remain for extended periods; 3 to 5 days is usually sufficient time for cure (along with concurrent antibiotics).[19]

Bile collections (sometimes called bilomas) from the liver are usually secondary to trauma, complications of liver transplantation, or secondary to a recent operation. Bile collections, as with any collections related to the liver, can be classified as (1) parenchymal (intrahepatic), (2) subcapsular, and (3) extrahepatic (subhepatic or suprahepatic/subphrenic). Subcapsular and extrahepatic collections are treated as any abdominal abscess drainage. However, intrahepatic/parenchymal bile collections (especially after liver transplantation) should be interrogated with contrast and fluoroscopy to assess communication with the biliary tract for both diagnostic and therapeutic

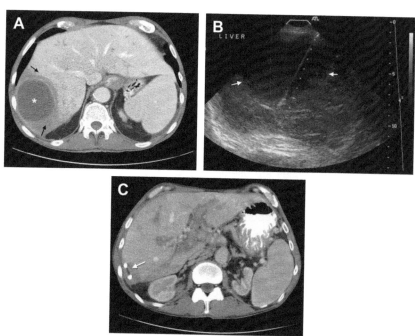

Fig. 10. Contrast-enhanced axial CT abdomen image (A) shows a large rim-enhancing low-density lesion consistent with an abscess (*white asterisk*) in the right hepatic lobe in a septic patient with obstructive jaundice secondary to hilar cholangiocarcinoma and marked perilesional edema (*black arrows*). (B) Placement of the drainage catheter into this intraparenchymal liver abscess (between *white arrows*) under ultrasound guidance. Contrast-enhanced axial CT abdomen image (C) shows complete resolution of the abscess with the pigtail catheter (*white arrow*) still in place. Also noted is dilatation of the intrahepatic biliary ducts.

purposes. Bilomas that communicate with the biliary tract usually require biliary drainage. Biliary drainage helps with reducing the reaccumulation of bile in the collection. Moreover, in liver transplants, the hepatic artery must be interrogated for hepatic arterial defects such as hepatic artery stenosis or thrombosis, which are common causes for parenchymal infarction, breakdown, and biloma formation (after the cavity necrosis into the biliary tract).

Echinococcal abscesses are endemic in certain areas worldwide (eg, Middle East, Greece, Argentina, New Zealand), but are uncommon in the United States. The diagnosis is based on the results of serologic testing. Percutaneous drainage is traditionally contraindicated because of concerns for the development of anaphylaxis and intraperitoneal spread. However, substantial experience has accumulated in the Middle East suggesting that these abscesses can usually be treated safely by percutaneous means.[20] If percutaneous drainage is to be entertained, a transhepatic drainage (not direct drainage in superficial echinococcal collections) is preferred. Furthermore, drainage of all the fluid is recommended, which is to be replaced with hyperosmolar saline in an attempt to kill the daughter cysts as soon as possible.

Splenic Abscesses

Splenic abscesses are even rarer than hepatic abscesses. Most are immunosuppression associated, are very small, and do not require catheter drainage. Posttraumatic superinfection of a hematoma is another cause of splenic abscess. Similarly, infected infarcts are seen in septicemic patients. Splenic cysts may become infected, and even the uncommon intrasplenic pancreatic pseudocyst may be infected. Considerations similar to those with other abscesses are useful and generally effective when treating splenic abscesses. However, large splenic abscesses may be treated with drainage.[21] Reports of successful drainage in infected hematomas after splenic salvage surgery have been published, in parallel with the increasingly conservative management of splenic trauma.[22]

Renal and Perirenal Abscesses

Renal and perirenal abscesses often are associated with pyelonephritis or nephrolithiasis and there may be hydronephrosis as well. As with hepatic and splenic abscesses, small renal abscesses may respond to antibiotics alone, whereas larger abscesses require drainage.[23,24] Septicemia is another cause of renal abscesses;

in this situation, the abscesses occasionally are multiple, bilateral, or both. Renal abscesses may rupture through the renal capsule into the perirenal space. These abscesses often are large. As with intrarenal abscesses, perirenal abscesses usually are amenable to percutaneous abscess drainage. If renal obstruction is associated with a renal or perirenal abscess, percutaneous nephrostomy may be needed for access to stone removal or to relieve a malignant or benign obstruction.

Pancreatic and Peripancreatic Abscesses

Pancreatic collections are diverse, and percutaneous options reflect the complexities of these collections. A standardized classification system has been developed for fluid collections associated with pancreatitis, in part to help guide therapy.[25] In general, acute collections are not infected. However, if superinfection of a peripancreatic fluid collection is suspected, percutaneous imaging-guided needle aspiration may be performed to obtain a specimen for culture. Infected pancreatic pseudocysts and pancreatic abscesses are generally drained routinely and urgently.[26-28] In contrast, noninfected asymptotic pancreatic pseudocysts may simply be observed in a substantial number of cases. Indications for drainage of noninfected pseudocysts include pain, imminent leak or rupture, and obstruction of the adjacent biliary or gastrointestinal tract by the pseudocyst.

Perhaps the major challenge with pancreatitis is the diagnosis and management of pancreatic necrosis. Pancreatic necrosis also may result in collections of material with the attenuation of fluid density on CT. This necrotic material (liquefied retroperitoneal fat) is viscous and often does not drain completely via a catheter. Large-caliber drainage catheters are usually required (at least 16F), and up to 22F to 24F catheters have been used by the current authors. If the area of necrosis is not infected, then the recommended treatment is supportive care. In some cases, the necrotic tissue liquefies and then becomes more amenable to catheter drainage.

Pancreatic abscesses are not seen until well into the course of pancreatitis, typically longer than 3 to 4 weeks. Multiple, complex collections often are present and require an adequate number and size of catheters. Pancreatic abscesses also occur after operating on the pancreas itself, such as with a partial pancreatectomy, or after operations on adjacent organs during which the pancreas is inadvertently injured. Another common surgery to cause pancreatic leak is splenectomy with inadvertent injury of the pancreatic tail. An occasional source of confusion with pancreatic collections is differentiation of a pancreatic pseudocyst from a cystic pancreatic tumor. The usual procedure of choice for these cystic tumors is surgical removal, although, on occasion, needle aspiration is performed because of an uncertain diagnosis or because of the compromised clinical status of the patient, and this may preclude operation.

COMPLICATIONS

Complications during percutaneous abscess drainage are rare and can be minimized with appropriate planning of the access route and daily rounding. Reported complication rates lie between none and 10% and are subject to variable definitions and thoroughness of reporting. Minor complications such as pain can be avoided by routine use of conscious sedation and adequate local anesthesia during catheter placement.

It is common for catheter drainage of an abscess to induce a bacteremia because abscess walls are highly vascular. Bacteremia may become clinical with new onset or exacerbation of sepsis. It is important to ensure that the patient has appropriate broad-spectrum antibiotic coverage before performing the abscess drainage. If the patient is not, then start the patient on intravenous ampicillin, gentamicin, and metronidazole before the procedure. When Gram stain and culture results become available, the antibiotic may be changed according to sensitivities. As with all interventional procedures, bleeding can occur, but its frequency can be reduced by correction of any coagulopathy before the procedure. Vascular injury may also occur from needles or catheters used to access abscesses. If the vessel is small, the bleeding usually stop spontaneously. A larger catheter may have to be inserted to tamponade the bleeding. If this does not work, angiographic embolization may be required. Bleeding may also occur because of associated oncotic pseudoaneurysms, which are more likely to occur from prior vascular surgeries or ramped inflammatory processes such as pancreatitis.

Percutaneous abscess drainage may be complicated by bowel perforation after being punctured by a needle, but in most cases there will be no sequela. Inadvertent catheter placement through the small bowel can be inconsequential and, when symptomatic, usually presents with high output of bowel contents from the catheter, which is easily recognized during clinical rounds. Alternatively, transenteric drainage may place the patient at risk for bowel obstruction. Inadvertent drainage through the colon places the patient at immediate risk for life-threatening peritonitis

and sepsis and warrants immediate surgical consultation. In all cases of transenteric catheter placement, if peritoneal signs are not present, consideration can be given to bowel rest, supportive care, and a course of broad-spectrum antibiotics. Withdrawal of the catheter without surgery is possible after a mature tract has developed, which can be verified by contrast-injection, over-the-wire tractogram.

Catheter placement through solid parenchymal organs can result in parenchymal, subcapsular, or peritoneal bleeding; vascular fistula formation; and pseudoaneurysm formation. These risks are minimal, as shown by literature studies describing percutaneous aspiration and drainage of abscesses located within the liver or spleen.[29–32] Most cases of catheter placement through solid parenchymal organs of the abdomen can be confirmed by CT and treated by catheter removal following adequate tract formation, or catheter removal with tract embolization using foam pledgets. Rare cases require transarterial embolization or surgery to treat hemorrhagic complications.

SUMMARY

Imaging-guided percutaneous drainage is a safe and effective treatment of abscesses. Interventional radiologists may use ultrasound, fluoroscopy, CT, or combined modalities for guidance of catheter placement in numerous locations in the abdomen and pelvis. After catheter placement, the performance of daily hospital rounds and the judicious use of follow-up imaging helps to optimize patient outcomes. Exchange or repositioning of the catheter, or insertion of an additional catheter, as well as adjuvant thrombolytic therapy, may be needed to achieve complete drainage.

REFERENCES

1. Ryan S, McGrath FP, Haslam PJ, et al. Ultrasound-guided endocavitary drainage of pelvic abscesses: technique, results and complications. Clin Radiol 2003;58:75–9.
2. Gerzof SG, Robbins AH, Johson WC, et al. Percutaneous catheter drainage of abdominal abscesses: five-year experience. N Engl J Med 1981;305:353–7.
3. Ferrucci JT, vanSonnenberg E. Intra-abdominal abscesses. Radiological diagnosis and treatment. JAMA 1981;246:2728–33.
4. vanSonnenberg E, Wittich GR, Goodacre BW, et al. Percutaneous abscess drainage: update [review]. World J Surg 2001;25(3):362–9 [discussion: 370–2].
5. Nolsøe CP, Torben L, Bjørn Ole S, et al. Interventional ultrasound. In: Dietrich CF, editor. London (UK): EFSUMB – European Course Book; 2011.

6. Gervais DA, Hahn PF, O'Neill MJ, et al. CT-guided transgluteal drainage of deep pelvic abscesses in children: selective use as an alternative to transrectal drainage. AJR Am J Roentgenol 2000;175:1393–6.

7. Haaga JR, Nakamoto D, Stellato T, et al. Intracavitary urokinase for enhancement of percutaneous abscess drainage: phase II trial. AJR Am J Roentgenol 2000;174:1681–5.

8. Dogra VS, Saad WE. Ultrasound-guided procedures. New York (NY): Thieme; 2009. p. 344.

9. Butch RJ, Mueller PR, Ferrucci JT, et al. Drainage of pelvic abscesses through the greater sciatic foramen. Radiology 1986;158:487–91.

10. Mueller PR, Simeone JF, Butch RJ, et al. Percutaneous drainage of subphrenic abscess: a review of 62 patients. AJR Am J Roentgenol 1986;147:1237–40.

11. McNicholas MM, Mueller PR, Lee MJ, et al. Percutaneous drainage of subphrenic fluid collections that occur after splenectomy: efficacy and safety of transpleural versus extrapleural approach. AJR Am J Roentgenol 1995;165:355–9.

12. Lee MJ, Wittich GR, Mueller PR. Percutaneous intervention in acute pancreatitis. Radiographics 1998;18:711–24.

13. Mueller PR, Ferrucci JT Jr, Simeone JF, et al. Lesser sac abscesses and fluid collections: drainage by transhepatic approach. Radiology 1985;155:615–8.

14. Shandera WX, Bollam P, Hashmey RH, et al. Hepatic amebiasis among patients in a public teaching hospital. South Med J 1998;91:829.

15. vanSonnenberg E, Mueller PR, Schiffman HR, et al. Intrahepatic amebic abscesses: indications for and results of percutaneous catheter drainage. Radiology 1985;156:631–5.

16. Ken JG, vanSonnenberg E, Casola G, et al. Perforated amebic liver abscesses: successful percutaneous treatment. Radiology 1989;170:195.

17. Tandon A, Jain AK, Dixit VK, et al. Needle aspiration in large amoebic liver abscess. Trop Gastroenterol 1997;18:19.

18. Moazam F, Nazir Z. Amebic liver abscess: spare the knife but save the child. J Pediatr Surg 1998;33:119.

19. Rajak CL, Gupta S, Jain S, et al. Percutaneous treatment of liver abscesses: needle aspiration versus catheter drainage. AJR Am J Roentgenol 1998;170:1035.

20. Filice C, Pirola F, Brunetti E, et al. A new therapeutic approach for hydatid liver cysts: aspiration and alcohol injection under sonographic guidance. Gastroenterology 1990;98:1366.

21. Rorbakken G, Schulz T. Splenic abscess caused by Salmonella braenderup, treated with percutaneous drainage and antibiotics. Scand J Infect Dis 1997;29:423–4.

22. Frumiento C, Sartorelli K, Vane D. Complications of splenic injuries: expansion of the nonoperative theorem. J Pediatr Surg 2000;35:788–91.

23. Wippermann CF, Schofer O, Beetz R, et al. Renal abscess in childhood: diagnostic and therapeutic progress. Pediatr Infect Dis J 1991;10:446–50.

24. Barker AP, Ahmed S. Renal abscess in childhood. Aust N Z J Surg 1991;61:217–21.

25. Bradley EL 3rd. A clinically based classification system for acute pancreatitis. Summary of the International Symposium on Acute Pancreatitis. Arch Surg 1993;128:586–90.

26. Mithofer K, Mueller PK, Warshaw AL. Interventional and surgical treatment of pancreatic abscess. World J Surg 1997;21:162.

27. vanSonnenberg E, Wittich GR, Casola G, et al. Percutaneous drainage of infected and noninfected pancreatic pseudocysts: experience in 101 cases. Radiology 1989;170:757.

28. vanSonnenberg E, Wittich GR, Chon KS, et al. Percutaneous radiologic drainage of pancreatic abscesses. AJR Am J Roentgenol 1997;168:979.

29. Chou YH, Hsu CC, Tiu CM, et al. Splenic abscess: sonographic diagnosis and percutaneous drainage or aspiration. Gastrointest Radiol 1992;17:262–6.

30. Do H, Lambiase RE, Deyoe L, et al. Percutaneous drainage of hepatic abscesses with and without intrahepatic biliary communication. AJR Am J Roentgenol 1991;157:1209–12.

31. Tazawa J, Sakai Y, Maekawa S, et al. Solitary and multiple pyogenic liver abscess: characteristics of the patients and efficacy of percutaneous drainage. Am J Gastroenterol 1997;92:271–4.

32. Gasparini D, Basadonna PT, DiDonna A. [Splenic abscesses: their percutaneous treatment and the role of the interventional radiologist]. Radiol Med 1994;87:803–7 [in Italian].

Ultrasound-Guided Visceral Biopsies: Renal and Hepatic

Nirvikar Dahiya, MD, William D. Middleton, MD,
Christine O. Menias, MD*

KEYWORDS

- Ultrasound • Biopsy • Renal • Hepatic • Perivascular • Pseudoaneurysm

KEY POINTS

- The basic approach to planning an ultrasound-guided biopsy is similar to performing any other interventional procedure.
- Visceral organ biopsies are being routinely done these days with excellent diagnostic results.
- Ultrasound is a safe and reliable imaging modality to provide guidance for the vast majority of biopsies.
- With good technique, these procedures have a very low complication rate.

 The authors have provided several related videos at http://www.ultrasound.theclinics.com/.

LIVER BIOPSY

Ultrasound-guided percutaneous biopsy of visceral organs in the abdomen has been in effect for many years. Paul Ehrlich is credited with performing the first percutaneous liver biopsy in 1883 in Germany.[1] Schüpfer[2] in 1907 published the first liver biopsy series. Huard and Baron popularized liver biopsy for general purposes in the1930s. Some of the more contemporary articles reporting ultrasound-guided procedures were written in 1972 by Goldberg and Pollack.[3] The basic approach to planning an ultrasound-guided biopsy is similar to performing any other interventional procedure. However, there are certain complexities specific to biopsy of the liver and kidney that are addressed in this article.

Indications for a Liver Biopsy

The indications for doing a liver biopsy are outlined in **Box 1**. A liver biopsy gives invaluable information regarding the staging, prognosis, and management even if clinical, laboratory, or imaging tests point to a specific focal or diffuse liver disease. Serial liver biopsies may help to monitor effects of specific therapy or to identify recurrence of disease.[4]

Preparation for a Liver Biopsy

The preparation of a liver biopsy constitutes the major portion of the work needed to execute a successful biopsy. The actual act of directing the needle to the target region and collecting the specimen only constitutes a small component of the procedure itself. A thorough history taking is imperative before the initiation of the biopsy. With this, the exact clinical question can be understood and the correct biopsy technique (fine-needle aspiration [FNA] vs core needle biopsy) determined; accordingly, the proper needle type and gauge can be selected. For instance, in patients with diffuse liver disease and a coexisting mass, it may be necessary to biopsy the mass (for diagnosis), the liver parenchyma (as part of preoperative surgical workup), or both depending

Section of Abdomen Imaging, Mallinckrodt Institute of Radiology, Washington University, 510 South Kingshighway, St Louis, MO 63110, USA
* Corresponding author.
E-mail address: meniasc@mir.wustl.edu

Ultrasound Clin 7 (2012) 363–375
doi:10.1016/j.cult.2012.03.004
1556-858X/12/$ – see front matter © 2012 Elsevier Inc. All rights reserved.

<table>
<tr><td>

Box 1
Indications for liver biopsy

Diffuse hepatocellular disease

Alcoholic liver disease

Nonalcoholic hepatic steatosis

Autoimmune hepatitis

Grading and staging of chronic hepatitis C or chronic hepatitis B

Heavy metal storage disorders such as hemochromatosis and Wilson disease

Cholestatic liver diseases such as primary biliary cirrhosis and primary sclerosing cholangitis

Abnormal liver function tests

Evaluation of efficacy or adverse effects of drugs such as methotrexate

Fever of unknown origin

Hepatosplenomegaly of unknown origin

Liver transplant rejection

Focal liver disease

Primary hepatocellular carcinoma,

Cholangiocarcinoma

Metastatic disease

Indeterminate mass

</td></tr>
</table>

or fresh frozen plasma can be considered dependent on the clinical evaluation. The decision to proceed can then be based on the location of the mass or the general condition of the patient.

Once the bleeding profile has been evaluated, it is important to review all the medications the patient is taking. Some patients may be on long-term anticoagulation or antiplatelet therapy, including aspirin, warfarin, clopidogrel bisulfate (PLAVIX; Bristol-Myers Squibb [New York, NY, USA]/Sanofi Pharmaceuticals [Bridgewater, NJ, USA]), and heparin. The referring physician must then determine if the risk of discontinuing the medicines is worse than the increased risk of bleeding related to the biopsy.

If the medications are to be discontinued, we follow the guidelines listed in **Table 1** to determine the period of time they are withheld. Regarding subcutaneous heparin, the liver biopsy can be performed if the PTT is within normal limits. Readers are advised to consult with their respective hematologic and clinical departments to ascertain guidelines for coagulation parameters and management of time for holding anticoagulants before doing a biopsy. Many times such decisions are made on a case-by-case basis.

An informed consent is obtained before proceeding with the biopsy. An allergy history to latex gloves and lidocaine is established at this time. All the steps of the procedure are explained to the patient in detail so that there are no surprises during the procedure itself.

Procedure of Doing the Liver Biopsy

A critical component of the procedure is choosing an approach for a liver biopsy. The ideal approach would be to find the shortest course to the target, avoiding lung, diaphragm, and all the vascular structures. However, this is not always possible. For a random liver biopsy, we prefer targeting the peripheral right hepatic lobe. This region is

on the clinical situation. In patients with multiple liver masses, prior workup may point to specific lesions that are worrisome and others that are clearly benign. If the patient had undergone positron emission tomography/computed tomography (PET-CT) as part of the workup, it is important to make a good anatomic correlation between the hypermetabolic lesion seen on the PET-CT and ultrasound examination. Some of the newer ultrasound equipments allow for fusion imaging, whereby an overlaying of the CT, magnetic resonance imaging, or PET can be done with the ultrasound examination to accurately identify the target.[5]

Once the clinical question has been understood, the prebiopsy workup includes evaluation of the bleeding profile of the patient and a detailed review of current medications taken by the patient. At our institution, we routinely obtain international normalized ratio (INR), platelet count, prothrombin time, and partial thromboplastin time (PTT). Our guidelines include performing a biopsy when INR is less than 1.5 and the platelet count is greater than 70,000/μL. Some institutions take a count of platelets of 50,000/μL as the minimum requirement.[6]

If the INR is greater than 1.5 or if the platelets are less than 70,000/μL, a transfusion of platelets and/

Table 1
Guidelines for management of anticoagulants before a visceral organ biopsy

Suggested Period of Discontinuity	Suggested Time Frame for Restarting Medication
Coumadin: 5–7 d	Resume the day of the procedure
Plavix: 7 d	Resume the next day
Ticlid: 10 d	Resume the next day
Heparin Drip: 6 h	Resume drip 12 h after procedure
Lovenox: 12 h	Resume 12 h after procedure

remote from the central hilar vasculature, and a tamponade effect can be achieved on completion of the biopsy by having the patient to lie in right lateral decubitus position. If a good subcostal window is available, it is our first preference. However, in most cases an intercostal approach is performed, in which the needle traverses the diaphragm and pleural space. Care should be taken to avoid the aerated lung. For this reason, we generally position the needle inferior to the transducer, so that shadowing from the lung can be visualized and avoided before the needle is advanced into the liver. When using the intercostal approach, the needle is directed over the ribs as the vascular bundle courses along the inferior edge of the ribs (**Fig. 1**).

A random biopsy of the left hepatic lobe is performed when the right hepatic lobe is not feasible. In most cases, the lateral section of the left lobe is targeted in a manner such that the left portal vein and artery can be avoided. Color Doppler is used as a mapping tool for all our biopsies.

Care is taken to minimize the risk of bleeding by trying to take the maximum length of the core tissue in the first pass. In cases in which the biopsy is of a target lesion within the liver, many have suggested choosing a biopsy path that courses through a part of the normal liver before reaching the target. Although there are no studies to prove it, this approach presumably helps with the tamponade effect if there is any bleeding from the target lesion after the biopsy (**Fig. 2**). It also may have a role in preventing seeding. We believe that there may be some justification to this approach, but we do not hesitate to biopsy lesions on the surface of the liver if they are substantially easier to reach than the deeper lesions.

Needles are categorized as aspiration- or suction-type needles (Menghini needle, Klatskin needle, Chiba needle, and Jamshidi needle) and cutting-type needles (Vim-Silverman needle and Tru-cut needle). The cutting-type needles can also be spring loaded. Most visceral core biopsies are now performed with spring-loaded needles. These needles can be further classified as side notch or end cutting (**Figs. 3–6**).

They can also be classified as automatic or semiautomatic. The semiautomatic needles allow one to manually advance the side-notch needle into the target. The biopsy is performed if the operator is satisfied with the placement of the notch in the target. The automatic needle obtains the core without providing the option of manual advancement. With this type of needle, it is critical to make accurate measurements of the target size to select an appropriate predefined length for core biopsy. The end-cutting needles used in our department yield full core specimens at lengths of 1.3, 2.3, or 3.3 cm, whereas the semiautomatic side-notch needle yields a partial core specimen at a length of 1 or 2 cm. This can vary depending on the biopsy device manufacturers. If the biopsy device that is chosen has a loud clicking sound while performing the procedure, it is best to make patients aware of this so that they do not get startled during the procedure when they hear the sound. In terms of guidance, the choice is between using a mechanical guide attached to the transducer and freehand guidance. The freehand technique requires more experience but has the distinct advantage of maneuverability, especially when subtle changes are required in direction or angle.

Choice of transducer used to guide the needle is also important. Provided visualization of the target and adjacent vessels is adequate, phased array transducers have many advantages because they are small and easy to maneuver, especially when using an intercostal approach. Linear array transducers provide the advantage of better

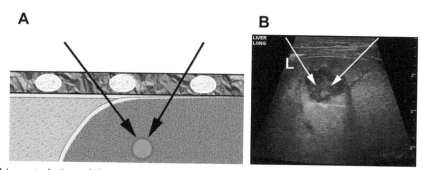

Fig. 1. Liver biopsy technique. (*A*) Longitudinal view of the liver and lung interface showing the potential danger of puncturing lung when performing biopsy via a superior approach. (*B*) Corresponding ultrasound image shows a bright reflection and dirty shadow arising from the aerated lung (L). Performing the biopsy from this trajectory risks potential lung puncture and pneumothorax. Arrows indicate the potential trajectories for liver mass biopsy.

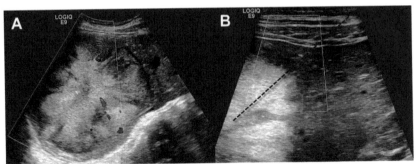

Fig. 2. Liver biopsy technique. (*A*) Transverse view of the right lobe of the liver showing a large liver metastasis. (*B*) Magnified high-resolution view of the medial aspect of the lesion showing a preferred needle trajectory to traverse normal liver parenchyma before entering the mass.

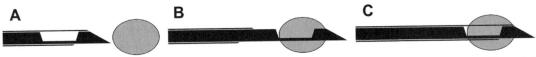

Fig. 3. Side-notch needle. (*A*) Side-notch needle in cocked position before biopsy of a focal lesion, (*B*) partially deployed position, and (*C*) fully deployed position.

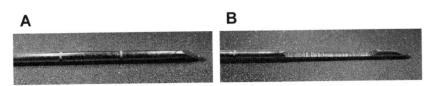

Fig. 4. Side-notch needles. (*A*) Side-notch needle in cocked position and (*B*) deployed position.

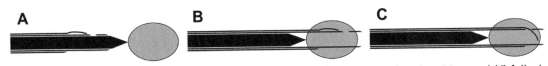

Fig. 5. Full-core needle. (*A*) Full-core needle in cocked position, (*B*) partially deployed position, and (*C*) fully deployed position.

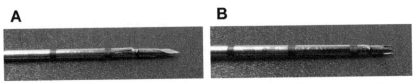

Fig. 6. Full-core needle. (*A*) Full-core needle in cocked position and (*B*) fully deployed position.

visualization if the target is superficial (ie, within approximately 5 cm of the skin surface). Curved array transducers provide an intermediate choice when lesions are too deep for a linear array, and visualization is inadequate with a phased array. The major disadvantage of curved arrays is their larger size, which makes them more clumsy to maneuver. Generally, we prefer lining up our biopsy needle along the side of the transducer, so that we can see the entire shaft of the needle as we approach the target (**Fig. 7**).

The sterile biopsy tray we use for a biopsy procedure includes

1. 10 mL of 1% lidocaine buffered with 8.4% sodium bicarbonate
2. 25-gauge × 30-mm needle
3. 4 × 4 gauze pack
4. Scalpel #11 blade
5. 5-mL syringe
6. 25-gauge × 5/8-in needle for superficial anesthesia
7. Applicator prep, gloves, and sterile drapes.

We perform most of our biopsies under local anesthesia, using 1% lidocaine mixed with sodium bicarbonate. The shorter 25-gauge × 5/8-in needle is used to inject lidocaine for superficial intradermal anesthesia after the patient has been cleaned and draped in a sterile manner. For deeper anesthesia, we use the 25-gauge × 30-mm needles to introduce more lidocaine. Deeper anesthesia is injected under ultrasound guidance to determine the proper trajectory for the biopsy and to ensure that the anesthesia is injected deep enough to numb the capsule of the viscera, be it the liver or the kidney.

Moderate sedation or conscious sedation is usually not necessary for routine liver biopsies; however, there are institutions that may typically use fentanyl (Sublimaze) and midazolam (Versed). If moderate sedation is used, special credentialing and privileging to perform sedation may be required.[7]

It helps to give a little extra 1% lidocaine at the capsule (**Fig. 8**). At times, it helps to inject enough so as to cause a slight bump in the contour of the parietal peritoneum; this serves as a landmark for the entry point of the biopsy needle.

Once the local anesthesia has been satisfactorily injected, we observe the relation between the biopsy target and the patient's breathing to determine if the biopsy will be done with the patient holding his/her breath in normal or deep inspiration or normal expiration. We usually ask the patient to practice a couple of breath-holds at this time to ascertain the best position of the target lesion for the biopsy. When possible, we prefer normal expiration because this is more reproducible than deep inspiration and it raises the location of lung parenchyma. However, this expiration may not be possible in patients who are short of breath.

For core biopsies, local anesthesia is followed by a small nick in the skin with a surgical blade. This is important because it can sometimes be difficult to advance core needles through the skin. The core needle we like to use is usually the spring-loaded 18-gauge needle. For liver biopsies, we most often use the end-cutting needle that yields a full core specimen at lengths of 1.3, 2.3, or 3.3 cm. When a focal lesion is near major vessels, a semiautomatic side-notch needle that yields a partial core specimen at a length of 1 or 2 cm may be preferable. In both cases, the needle is introduced to the capsule surface; patients are then asked to hold their breath and the needle is

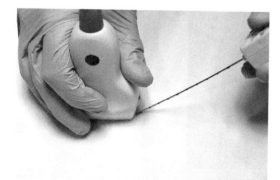

Fig. 7. Freehand biopsy technique. Biopsy needle is positioned in the plane of the image, immediately next to the side of the transducer. This allows for visualization of the needle tip and shaft throughout the procedure.

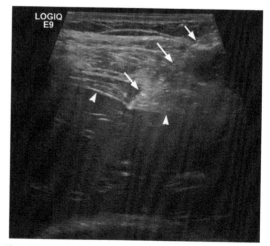

Fig. 8. Liver capsule numbing. Needle shaft and tip (*arrows*) are positioned such that anesthesia administered is at the level of the liver capsule (*arrowheads*).

introduced into the liver. In most cases, if the trajectory has been well planned and the needle is well visualized, the needle can be advanced to the lesion and a sample can be obtained on a single breath-hold.

The throw of the needle depends on the location and size of the lesion and the distribution of adjacent vessels. It is important, however, to remember that a throw setting of 10 or 13 mm typically results in a sample that is several millimeters shorter. So, if safe, it is best to avoid these short throws. For random liver biopsies, we mostly use the 3.3-cm throw.

For FNA, we use either a 25-gauge spinal needle or a 23-gauge Chiba needle. In both cases, we prefer introducing the needle with the stylet inside to avoid contaminating the lumen with extraneous cells and to ensure that the needle has some tensile strength to maneuver. Once the needle tip has reached the target, the stylet can be removed and the process of taking the FNA sample can begin (**Fig. 9**). Typically, we do the first aspiration without suction. Subsequent aspirations are performed with or without suction depending on the yield of the initial pass. Although we prefer making multiple separate passes, sometimes successful and consistent needle placement may be very difficult.

In these cases, coaxial technique can be performed,[7] wherein an introducer is initially deployed into the target area and subsequent sampling can be done coaxially through it. Although a distinct advantage of the coaxial technique is the single puncture through the liver capsule, it is somewhat offset by the increased risk of capsule shearing or tearing as the needle stays in for a longer period while the patient breathes.

The choice of performing an FNA biopsy or a core biopsy depends on the clinical scenario. In a patient with a known extrahepatic primary cancer in whom the only reason to perform a liver biopsy is to prove the presence of metastatic disease, we would do an FNA. If immediate on-site cytologic analysis is possible, aspirations are performed until a diagnostic sample is obtained. If the initial aspiration result is positive for malignancy and correlates with the primary tumor, no additional aspirations are required. If the initial specimens are negative for malignancy or suggest an alternative primary, then additional aspirations or core biopsies are obtained. If only semi-immediate off-site cytologic analysis is possible or if there is no cytologic support, several passes (3–6) should be obtained before terminating the procedure.

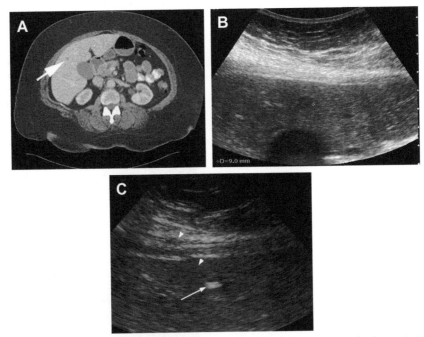

Fig. 9. FNA. A 55-year-old woman with a history of pancreatic cancer. Small liver mass in the patient with a history of pancreatic cancer and a suspicious lesion seen on CT. (*A*) Contrast-enhanced CT scan of the liver showing a small low-attenuation lesion in the liver (*arrow*). (*B*) Transverse sonogram of the liver shows a 9-mm solid hypoechoic lesion (*cursors*) corresponding to the lesion seen on CT. (*C*) Image obtained from a real-time cine clip taken during FNA shows the tip of a 25-gauge spinal needle (*arrow*) within the lesion. Needle shaft location (*arrowheads*) was more apparent during real-time imaging.

Despite the presence of a known extrahepatic primary tumor, if immunohistochemical studies are anticipated, we typically do a core biopsy rather than an FNA. A core biopsy provides enough tissue for hematoxylin-eosin as well as immunohistochemical staining. Additional sections can be taken from the paraffin block of the core biopsy to stain for immunohistochemistry markers such as estrogen receptor, progesterone receptor, and HER2/neu.

If the clinical history or prior imaging results suggest a primary malignant or benign liver tumor, we generally perform core biopsies with an 18-gauge needle (**Fig. 10**).

If hepatocellular cancer is confirmed, it is permissible to start with FNA and get preliminary analysis from the respective cytopathologist. If the diagnosis of hepatocellular cancer is confirmed after 1 to 3 passes, no further aspirations are necessary. But if the initial aspiration results are negative or nondiagnostic, cores become necessary. In patients with suspected hepatocellular cancer and tumor thrombus of the portal or hepatic vein, it is possible to confirm the diagnosis and assist with staging by performing FNA of the tumor thrombus.[8] At times, referring hepatologists do not require a tissue diagnosis to confirm the presence of hepatocellular carcinoma if the cross-sectional imaging is consistent with hepatocellular carcinoma and there is a correlative elevation of α-fetoprotein level.

The diagnostic accuracy of percutaneous needle biopsy in lesions 1 cm or smaller has increased from 79% (n = 24) in 1987 to 87.5% (n = 24) in 1993 and 99% (n = 74) in 1999. The use of a free-hand biopsy technique under ultrasound guidance is a common feature of all the series.[9]

Complications

Liver biopsies are relatively safe, with a complication rate of 0.2% to 0.3%.[10] Hemorrhage is the most common complication and is more likely to occur in patients with underlying cirrhosis or malignancy or bleeding diathesis. Most complications occur soon after completion of the biopsy. A linear color flow signal may at times be seen along the needle track immediately after the biopsy.[11] Kim and colleagues[11] evaluated the predictive role this signal played in the detection of postbiopsy

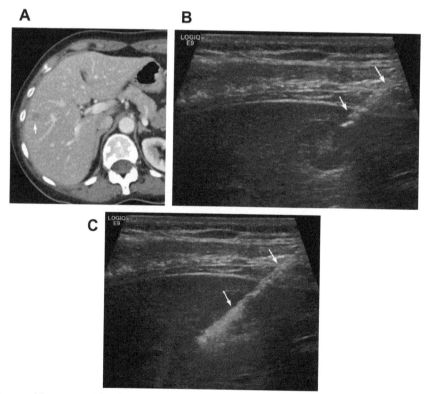

Fig. 10. A 61-year-old woman with a history of breast cancer. (*A*) Contrast-enhanced CT scan shows a small superficial low-attenuation lesion in the right lobe of the liver (*arrow*). (*B*) Oblique ultrasound image shows an 18-gauge core needle (*arrows*) in position to obtain a core biopsy. (*C*) The needle is deployed (*arrows*) and traverses the entire diameter of the lesion. Note that the throw in this case was selected at 20 mm to ensure sampling of the entire lesion.

bleeding and referred to it as patent track sign. The investigators suggested that the postbiopsy bleeding events were significantly more likely when a patent track sign persisted on scans obtained 5 minutes after the biopsy (**Fig. 11**).

Ascites should not be considered a contraindication to liver biopsy; however, in cases of moderate to large ascites, we prefer to have a paracentesis done before the biopsy. In cases in which patients are affected by significant coagulopathy, we recommend a transjugular hepatic biopsy.

RENAL BIOPSY

Percutaneous renal biopsy using an aspiration needle and with the patient in sitting position was first described by Iversen and Brun[12] in 1951. In 1954, Kark and Muehrcke[13] described the use of the cutting Vim-Silverman needle in patients in the prone position, with a substantial improvement in the rate of success. The 1961 Ciba Foundation Symposium on renal biopsy marked the coming of age of this technique.[14] Recent advances in

imaging, interventional, and cytologic techniques have enhanced the role of percutaneous biopsy in the diagnosis of renal masses. The incidental detection of benign and malignant renal masses has increased with increase in use of multidetector CT and magnetic resonance imaging.[15]

In one study, 25% of masses smaller than 3 cm were benign.[16] This factor has led to an increased demand for percutaneous renal biopsies for smaller masses. Biopsy of oncocytoma has been controversial. The reason lies in the difficulty presented to differentiate benign cells from malignant cells on pathologic examination. Oncocytic cells can exist in various renal neoplasms, including renal oncocytoma and oncocytic renal cell carcinomas, many of which are renal cell carcinomas of low metastatic potential.[17] These include granular cell carcinoma, chromophobe renal cell carcinoma, and eosinophilic variant of papillary renal cell carcinoma.[18–21] In some cases, a diagnosis of oncocytoma can be strongly suggested on the basis of histochemical, immunocytochemical, and ultrastructural studies. Oncocytomas could

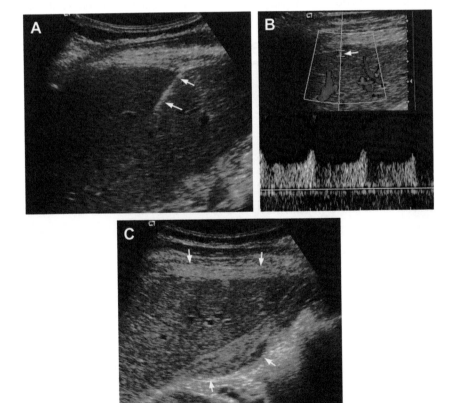

Fig. 11. A 60-year-old man with chronic hepatitis C referred for an ultrasound-guided random liver biopsy. (*A*) Oblique view of the liver shows the core needle (*arrows*) in position obtaining a random liver biopsy. (*B*) Postbiopsy scan shows a patent tract (*arrow*) with detectable Doppler signal at the biopsy site. (*C*) Postbiopsy image obtained 2 hours after the procedure shows an acute hematoma surrounding the liver (*arrows*). This required Gelfoam embolization by an interventional radiologist.

be confidently distinguished from oncocytic renal cell carcinoma using immunocytochemical analysis. In a study done by Liu and Fanning,[22] all oncocytomas were negative for vimentin, whereas only granular cell carcinoma and eosinophilic variant of papillary renal cell carcinoma were positive for vimentin. Also, the 2 vimentin-negative neoplasms, oncocytoma and chromophobe renal cell carcinoma, could be distinguished by Hale colloidal iron stain, which was present in all chromophobe renal cancers but only focally or not at all in oncocytomas.

Indications for a Renal Biopsy

As with the liver, kidney biopsies may be done either to evaluate an indeterminate focal lesion/mass or to evaluate the cortex for a parenchymal disease process. A list of the more important indications is presented in **Box 2**.

Preparation for Renal Biopsy

The issues related to preparation for the biopsy have already been discussed in the liver biopsy section and are essentially the same. The coagulation workup and the assessment for medications that interfere with clotting mechanisms are also similar. The fundamental difference comes in the approach to a kidney biopsy and the associated complications. As with hepatic biopsies, renal biopsies, whether focal or nonfocal, can be performed as outpatient procedures under ultrasound guidance.

Box 2
Indications for renal biopsy

Parenchymal renal disease

Nephrotic syndrome

Isolated glomerular hematuria

Systemic disease with renal dysfunction

Acute nephritic syndrome

Unexplained acute renal failure

Goodpasture syndrome

Wegener granulomatosis

Suspected renal transplant rejection

Solitary renal mass for which partial nephrectomy may be considered

Multiple renal masses

Renal mass in a patient with a known primary malignancy or metastatic disease or lymphoma

Renal mass in a patient with potential focal infection/abscess

---

Focal mass lesion biopsy

For focal biopsies of a mass lesion, FNA and core biopsy can both be performed. Some institutions may perform both in the same sitting because a combination of the two may produce higher diagnostic yield. Whereas FNA may be performed using a 22- or 25-gauge needle, 18-gauge needles are used for core biopsies. We do 4 to 6 passes for our FNA samples and 2 or more samples for our core biopsies. The patient is put in a posterior oblique or lateral decubitus position for most biopsies. A towel or pillow may be put between the body and the bed to enhance the kyphosis. This helps in pushing the rib cage up and increasing the space available for doing the biopsy. We try to use the posterior axillary line as the point of entry. This posterolateral approach avoids the potential inadvertent injury to the colon. Sometimes the location of the mass may prompt a more posterior approach in prone position (**Fig. 12**). Once the mass has been visualized using ultrasound, anesthesia is administered in a manner similar to that described for liver biopsies.

Nonfocal renal cortex (cortical) biopsy

Nonfocal parenchymal biopsies are performed in whatever position provides optimal visualization of the kidney and avoids critical overlying structures. The lower pole of either kidney is the preferred site. Usually the left kidney is the first choice because it is lower in location than the right. The target is the cortical tissue from the lower pole of the kidney. Care is taken to avoid the medulla and the collecting system by directing the needle into the superficial cortex in a relatively tangential manner. An onsite pathology service determines the adequacy of the sample (**Fig. 13**).

Complications

Renal biopsy is a relatively safe procedure, with loss of life extremely rare and major complications, mostly related to bleeding, occurring in only 1% to 6% of procedures.[23] Renal biopsies have an overall low mortality rate of 0.031%.[24]

Postbiopsy complications include hemorrhage, pseudoaneurysm, arteriovenous fistula, infection, pneumothorax, adjacent bowel or liver/spleen injury, and tumor seeding. Postbiopsy bleeding can occur in several places: into the collecting system, leading to microscopic or gross hematuria and possible ureteral obstruction; in a subcapsular location, leading to pressure tamponade and pain; or into the perinephric space, leading to retroperitoneal hematoma and possibly a drop in the serum hematocrit level (**Fig. 14**). Most clinically

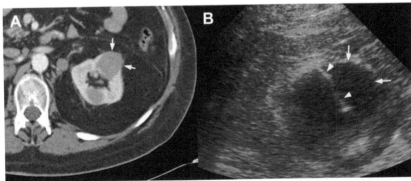

Fig. 12. A 24-year-old man with a history of lymphoma. (*A*) Contrast-enhanced CT scan shows a low-attenuation lesion in the anterior aspect of the left kidney (*arrows*). Other similar lesions were seen in both kidneys. (*B*) Transverse sonogram showing an 18-gauge core needle (*arrowheads*) within a hypoechoic solid renal mass (*arrows*) corresponding to the lesion shown on CT. Pathology from this biopsy was consistent with lymphoma.

significant bleedings are recognized within 12 to 24 hours of the biopsy.[25]

Mild perinephric hemorrhage is self-limiting and seen in 44% of the cases.[26] If there is a large retroperitoneal hematoma, the patient will have to be closely monitored and may even need other imaging modalities to assess the extent of bleed.

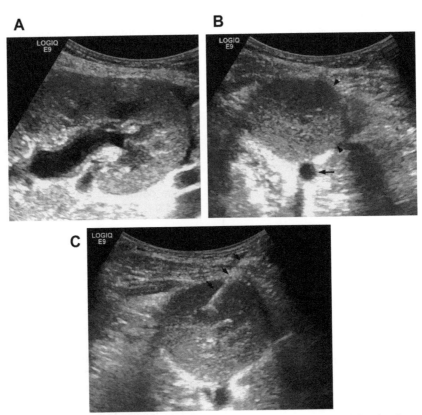

Fig. 13. Status after renal transplant in a 45-year-old woman with elevated creatinine levels and concern for rejection. (*A*) Longitudinal view of the lower pole of the transplant. Identification of cortex without calyces and medullary components is important. (*B*) Transverse view of the lower pole of the transplant (*arrowheads*) shows the relationship of the transplant with the external iliac artery (*arrow*). (*C*) Transverse view with needle in position showing the eccentric oblique orientation of the needle (*arrows*) used to obtain cortical tissue with little or no medullary component.

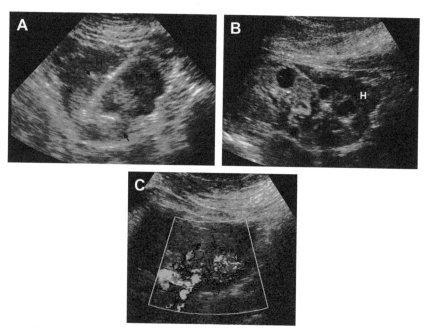

Fig. 14. A 60-year-old woman with parenchymal renal disease referred for a percutaneous biopsy. (*A*) Transverse view of the lower pole of the kidney obtained during performance of a second core biopsy shows a hypoechoic perinephric hematoma (H). The core needle is shown within the lower pole of the more echogenic kidney (*arrows*). (*B*) Longitudinal view following both biopsies again shows the perinephric hematoma (H). (*C*) Color Doppler view of the lower pole of the left kidney shows extensive perivascular tissue vibration (*arrows*) consistent with an arteriovenous fistula.

Pseudoaneurysm and arteriovenous fistula formation are also well-recognized complications of percutaneous renal biopsy (**Fig. 15**). They can be clinically silent, or the patient may present with hematuria or retroperitoneal bleeding. Color duplex Doppler and CT angiography are both sensitive for making the diagnosis. In some cases arterial embolization may be required.[27,28] Tumor seeding is always a theoretical possibility; however, only 7 cases have been reported in the literature.[27–34]

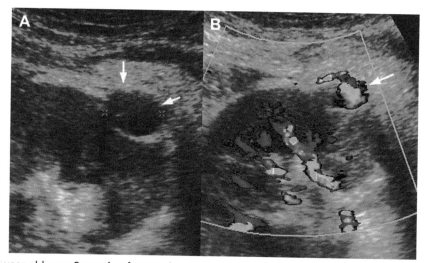

Fig. 15. A 66-year-old man, 8 months after renal transplant with pain one day after renal biopsy. (*A*) Longitudinal view of the lower pole of the transplant shows a hypoechoic perinephric lesion (*arrows*). (*B*) Color Doppler image confirms internal vascular flow. An arterial signal was documented on waveform analysis consistent with a perinephric pseudoaneurysm (*arrow*).

POSTBIOPSY CARE

We observe patients after a liver or renal biopsy for at least 4 hours. After a baseline assessment of vital signs in the department, the patients are observed in the postanesthesia care unit. Pulse rate, blood pressure, and oxygen saturation are monitored. Some patients will have local tenderness once the effect of lidocaine wears off, which can be symptomatically treated with a variety of analgesics. Some patients complain of right shoulder pain after a liver biopsy. This is likely a viscerosomatic referred pain[35] and is self-limiting. Right shoulder pain does not seem to be an indication of a severe complication such as intra-abdominal bleeding.[36]

If the patients complain of severe pain at the site of the biopsy or if the blood pressure falls, they are brought back to the department to assess the biopsy site by ultrasonography. Rarely a patient may need a CT scan if concerns for a more severe hepatic or renal injury are high. Patients without complaints are discharged with instructions to avoid strenuous activity for the remaining day.

SUMMARY

Visceral organ biopsies are being routinely done these days with excellent diagnostic results. Ultrasonography is a safe and reliable imaging modality to provide guidance for the vast majority of biopsy. With good technique, these procedures have a very low complication rate.

SUPPLEMENTARY DATA

Supplementary data related to this article can be found online at doi:10.1016/j.cult.2012.03.004.

REFERENCES

1. van Leeuwen DJ, Wilson L, Crowe DR. Liver biopsy in the mid-1990s: questions and answers. Semin Liver Dis 1995;15:340–59.
2. Schüpfer F. De la possibilite de faire "intra vitam" un diagnostic histo-pathologique précis des maladies due foie et de la rate. Sem Med 1907;27:229 [in French].
3. Goldberg BB, Pollack HM. Ultrasonic aspiration transducer. Radiology 1972;102:187–9.
4. Bravo AA, Sheth SG, Chopra S. Current concepts: liver biopsy. N Engl J Med 2001;7:495–500.
5. Krücker J, Xu S, Venkatesan A, et al. Clinical utility of real-time fusion guidance for biopsy and ablation. J Vasc Interv Radiol 2011;22(4):515–24.
6. Khati NJ, Gorodenker J, Hill MC. Ultrasound-guided biopsies of the abdomen. Ultrasound Q 2011;27(4): 255–68.
7. Winter TC, Lee FT Jr, Hinshaw JL. Ultrasound-guided biopsies in the abdomen and pelvis. Ultrasound Q 2008;24(1):45–68.
8. Tarantino L, Francica G, Sordelli I, et al. Diagnosis of benign and malignant portal vein thrombosis in cirrhotic patients with hepatocellular carcinoma: color Doppler US, contrast-enhanced US, and fine-needle biopsy. Abdom Imaging 2006;31:537–44.
9. Yu SC, Liew CT, Lau WY, et al. US-guided percutaneous biopsy of small (≤1-cm) hepatic lesions. Radiology 2001;218:195–9.
10. Piccinino F, Sagnelli E, Pasquale G, et al. Complications following percutaneous liver biopsy. A multicentre retrospective study on 68,276 biopsies. J Hepatol 1986;2(2):165.
11. Kim KW, Kim MJ, Kim HC, et al. Value of "patent track" sign on Doppler sonography after percutaneous liver biopsy in detection of postbiopsy bleeding: a prospective study in 352 patients. Am J Roentgenol 2007;189(1):109–16.
12. Iversen P, Brun C. Aspiration biopsy of the kidney. Am J Med 1951;11:324–30.
13. Kark RM, Muehrcke RC. Biopsy of kidney in prone position. Lancet 1954;266:1047–9.
14. Wolstenholme GE, Cameron MP, Ciba Foundation. Ciba Foundation Symposium on Renal Biopsy: clinical and pathological significance. London: J Churchill; 1961.
15. Silverman SG, Gan YU, Koenraad J, et al. Imaging-guided percutaneous renal biopsy: rationale and approach. AJR Am J Roentgenol 2010;194(6): 1443–9.
16. Frank I, Blute ML, Cheville JC, et al. Solid renal tumors: an analysis of pathological features related to tumor size. J Urol 2003;170:2217–20.
17. Krejci KG, Blute ML, Cheville JC, et al. Nephron-sparing surgery for renal cell carcinoma: clinico-pathologic features predictive of patient outcome. Urology 2003;62:641–6.
18. Wiatrowska BA, Zakowski MF. Fine-needle aspiration biopsy of chromophobe renal cell carcinoma and oncocytoma: comparison of cytomorphologic features. Cancer 1999;87:161–7.
19. Akhtar M, Ali MA. Aspiration cytology of chromophobe cell carcinoma of the kidney. Diagn Cytopathol 1995;13:287–94.
20. Alanen KA, Tyrkko JE, Nurmi MJ. Aspiration biopsy cytology of renal oncocytoma. Acta Cytol 1985;29: 859–62.
21. Granter SR, Renshaw AA. Fine-needle aspiration of chromophobe renal cell carcinoma: analysis of six cases. Cancer 1997;81:122–8.
22. Liu J, Fanning CV. Can renal oncocytomas be distinguished from renal cell carcinoma on fine-needle aspiration specimens? A study of conventional smears in conjunction with ancillary studies. Cancer 2001;93:390–7.

23. Korbet SM. Percutaneous renal biopsy. Semin Nephrol 2002;22:254–67.

24. Smith EH. Complications of percutaneous abdominal fine-needle biopsy. Radiology 1991;178:253–8.

25. Whittier WL, Korbet SM. Timing of complications in percutaneous renal biopsy. J Am Soc Nephrol 2004;15(1):142.

26. Lechevallier E, André M, Barriol D, et al. Fine needle percutaneous biopsy with computerized tomography guidance. Radiology 2000;216:506–10.

27. Abe M, Saitoh M. Selective renal tumor biopsy under ultrasonic guidance. Br J Urol 1992;70:7–11.

28. Silberzweig JE, Tey S, Winston JA, et al. Percutaneous renal biopsy complicated by renal capsular artery pseudoaneurysm. Am J Kidney Dis 1998;31:533–5.

29. Gibbons RP, Bush WH Jr, Burnett LL. Needle tract seeding following aspiration of renal cell carcinoma. J Urol 1977;118:865–7.

30. Auvert J, Abbou CC, Lavarenne V. Needle tract seeding following puncture of renal oncocytoma. Prog Clin Biol Res 1982;100:597–8.

31. Kiser GC, Totonchy M, Barry JM. Needle tract seeding after percutaneous renal adenocarcinoma aspiration. J Urol 1986;136:1292–3.

32. Wehle MJ, Grabstald H. Contraindications to needle aspiration of a solid renal mass: tumor dissemination by renal needle aspiration. J Urol 1986;136:446–8.

33. Shenoy PD, Lakhkar BN, Ghosh MK, et al. Cutaneous seeding of renal carcinoma by Chiba needle aspiration biopsy: case report. Acta Radiol 1991;32:50–2.

34. Slywotzky C, Maya M. Needle tract seeding of transitional cell carcinoma following fine-needle aspiration of a renal mass. Abdom Imaging 1994;19:174–6.

35. Hartmann H, Beckh K. Nerve supply and nervous control of liver function. sections 1–13. In: McIntyre N, Benhamou JP, Bircher J, editors. Oxford textbook of clinical hepatology, vol. 1. Oxford (UK): Oxford University Press; 1993. p. 93.

36. Eisenberg E, Konopniki M, Veitsman E, et al. Prevalence and characteristics of pain induced by percutaneous liver biopsy. Anesth Analg 2003;96(5):1392–6.

Percutaneous and Intra-operative Tumor Ablation

Jonathan K. West, MD[a], Minhaj S. Khaja, MD, MBA[a],*,
Maryam Ashraf, MA[b], Wael E. Saad, MBBCh, FSIR[c]

KEYWORDS

- Tumor ablation • Intra-operative • Radiofrequency ablation • RFA • Cryoablation

KEY POINTS

- Percutaneous and intra-operative ablation procedures may offer curative or bridging, minimally invasive treatments to patients who are unable to undergo surgical resection for local tumor control.
- Careful preprocedural patient evaluation and postprocedural management are imperative in obtaining positive treatment results.
- Percutaneous tumor ablative therapies have shown efficacy in local tumor control in a variety of organs and tumor types, most commonly within the liver and kidneys.

INTRODUCTION

The past 2 decades have brought with them significant technological development and advancement in image-guided tumor ablation. The drive for this development is the discovery and application of minimally invasive methods to treat solid tumors locally without adjacent tissue damage. This strategy allows clinicians to broaden the patient population eligible for curative treatment and reduce morbidity and mortality associated with tumor resection. Tumors are now commonly treated with percutaneous and intra-operative (mostly laparoscopic) ablative therapies, especially in the liver and kidneys. Despite nuances in techniques, ablation is generally accomplished via placement of probes into the tissue of concern and induction of local cell death via various ablative mechanisms. Chemical ablation, such as direct tumor injection with ethanol or acetic acid, has largely been supplanted by thermal ablative techniques.[1] Many different technologies are available for ablation, including specialized probe technology and various methods of image guidance.

Thermal ablation can be accomplished by using probes that generate heat from radiofrequency (RF), microwaves, laser, or focused ultrasound, or alternatively by probes that cool tissues to lethal temperatures, called cryoablation. These ablative technologies have been extensively used over the past decade and have shown favorable results for minimally invasive destruction of focal solid tumors with relatively low morbidity and mortality, especially in individuals who are not operative candidates or do not wish to undergo surgical resection.[1,2] The goal of tumor ablation is to destroy all tumor cells in a mass as well as malignant cells adjacent to the visible tumor. As a result, the ablative therapy should include a 1-cm margin surrounding the target mass.[3] This strategy must be balanced with attempts to preserve surrounding normal tissue.

RF ablation (RFA) is the most commonly used and studied form of tumor ablation. Thus, we focus our discussion on RFA and only briefly discuss cryoablation. Other ablative methods are beyond the scope of this text and are not discussed. This article reviews the indications, preprocedural

[a] Division of Vascular and Interventional Radiology, Radiology and Medical Imaging, University of Virginia Health System, Charlottesville, VA, USA; [b] Graduate School of Arts & Sciences, University of Virginia, PO Box 400781, Charlottesville, VA 22904, USA; [c] Division of Vascular Interventional Radiology, Department of Radiology and Imaging Sciences, University of Virginia Health System, Charlottesville, VA, USA
* Corresponding author.
E-mail address: msk9f@virginia.edu

Ultrasound Clin 7 (2012) 377–397
doi:10.1016/j.cult.2012.03.003
1556-858X/12/$ – see front matter Published by Elsevier Inc.

patient evaluation, techniques, postprocedural management, and complications of ultrasound-guided percutaneous and intra-operative tumor ablation, with special attention to hepatic and renal neoplasms.

PLANNING AND PREPROCEDURAL CONSIDERATIONS

All patients undergoing tumor ablation with ultrasound guidance should be evaluated with a complete history and physical examination, and special attention should be paid to history of bleeding disorders, reactions or allergies to sedative or anesthetic medications, body habitus, and ability to position the patient appropriately (ie, patients unable to lie flat because of heart failure require a more specific plan). Each patient's comorbidities should be considered in addition to the possibilities of multiple tumors being present and the functional reserve of the organ of interest. Before a therapeutic ablation, the patient should have a full imaging and pathologic diagnostic workup. Often with liver, renal, or adrenal masses, cross-sectional imaging with intravenous contrast is performed for diagnostic evaluation and preprocedural planning purposes. In addition to aiding in diagnosis, the imaging allows for visualization of the patient's relevant anatomy and planning of approach with a necessary evaluation of intervening structures such as bowel. Diagnostic ultrasonography before the procedure also helps in evaluating how well the lesion can be seen with ultrasound during the forthcoming procedure. Biopsy before ablation may be performed but is controversial and may not be necessary in some settings in which history and imaging point to a specific diagnosis. Occasionally, small tissue samples can come back with inconclusive pathologic results and cloud the clinical picture.

Preoperative laboratory evaluation is necessary before the ablation procedure. Most importantly, a coagulation panel helps to rule out bleeding disorders. Complete blood counts establish a baseline hematocrit and white blood cell count to monitor for bleeding or infection if there are signs of complication. A platelet count of greater than 50 to 70,000/mm^3 and an international normalized ratio less than 1.4 are commonly used guidelines followed by many institutions. In addition, bilirubin values less than 3 mg/dL help rule out hepatic failure or obstructive jaundice.[4] These parameters have not been validated specifically, but rather represent a reflection of commonly used guidelines and operator comfort levels. The operator must consider the risks and benefits of the procedure. Metabolic panels, which include liver function tests for liver tumor ablation and creatinine for renal tumor

ablations, are helpful to establish baseline values to monitor recovery after the procedure. Obtaining tumor markers such as α-fetoprotein and carcinoembryonic antigen may be helpful in monitoring response in patients with hepatocellular carcinoma (HCC) or colorectal metastasis, respectively. Prophylactic antibiotics should be given within an hour before the procedure.[5]

Tumor size, location, and characteristics are important in preprocedural planning and should be thoroughly addressed. Specifics regarding different tumors and organs are discussed in later sections. In general, tumors must be locally confined, the target must be clear, and sizes greater than 3 to 4 cm are significantly more complicated to treat and usually require multiple sessions to obtain a 0.5-cm to 1-cm ablation margin.[4]

We prefer general anesthesia especially in complicated cases, patients with low pain tolerance and high level of anxiety, large lesions, or when precise breath control is required. Procedures should ideally be performed in a dedicated procedure/operating room with capabilities for endotracheal intubation and appropriate monitoring equipment. Standard surgical sterile technique should be followed by the entire staff involved.[5]

PATIENT AND TREATMENT MODALITY SELECTION

Correct patient selection is critical in planning ablative therapies. Details for specific indications in the liver, kidney, and adrenals are explained in their respective sections later. Increased tumor size carries with it increased risk of complication and risk of leaving behind residual disease. If the tumor location is adjacent to vital structures, careful consideration must be made to approach the areas of concern, and protective measures taken to insulate them. Centrally located tumors generally have larger nearby vessels, resulting in more of a heat-sink effect, and often have more adjacent vital structures that can be injured, such as the biliary tree in the liver or the urinary collecting system in the kidney.

When choosing an ablation modality, all of the factors mentioned earlier must be considered. RFA has the advantage of being the most well studied and likely the most familiar modality for most operators. RFA has an inherent cautery effect on small blood vessels, low cost, and quick ablation times (<20 minutes). Large nearby vessels can create a heat sink and protect a nearby tumor or reduce effective ablation area. RFA is more painful than cryoablation and less effective in treating cystic lesions. Cryoablation has longer procedure times (>25 minutes) and increased cost, but inherent anesthetic properties. Ablation is precise using cryoprobes because the ice-ball can be watched in real time, multiple probes can be used simultaneously for formation of larger ice-balls, and each probe can be individually controlled.[6] Some studies suggest that cryoablation causes less damage to the collecting system and bile ducts. The probe tract cannot be ablated with cryoablation, which theoretically increases the risk of tumor seeding and bleeding. This bleeding risk is less in the kidney when compared with the liver, because hemorrhage should be tamponaded by Gerota's fascia. Cryoablation seems to be less susceptible to the cold-sink effect of nearby vessels and more readily overcomes this effect, thereby allowing for ablation of perivascular tumor. Fibrous or spindle cell neoplasms have less water content and may be more resistant to cryoablation.[7]

TECHNIQUE AND PROBE TECHNOLOGY

Using ultrasound for real-time guidance to the target, ablation probe placement is similar to the technique used for percutaneous biopsy procedures using the direct trocar technique. When planning the approach, cross-sectional imaging must be examined in detail to avoid traversing vital organs during the procedure. Ideally, a path should be chosen that avoids the pleural space, gastrointestinal tract, and vessels. Some operators drain ascites, because it is believed that ascites prevents tamponade of bleeding. Details regarding technique are described later in reference to hepatic tumor ablation (including figures). Renal tumor RFA is similar and key differences are also discussed.

After appropriate general anesthesia is obtained, the preplanned path is illustrated with ultrasound, using a 4-MHz to 5-MHz multiarray transducer. The target lesion is identified, taking care to recognize any positional changes that may affect the pathway to the target (ie, intervening bowel). A planning ultrasound scan should also assess for tumor growth or increase in lesion number. When selecting a path, a peripheral segment of normal hepatic parenchyma should be crossed before entering the tumor if possible.[8] We prefer to mark the skin and outline the transducer, which aids in properly preparing and draping the patient (**Fig. 1**). The patient is then prepared in a sterile fashion with chlorhexidine and a sterile, fenestrated drape. The operator should be scrubbed and in sterile surgical attire (gown, gloves, and mask with eye protection) (**Fig. 2**). Local anesthetic (1% lidocaine) is

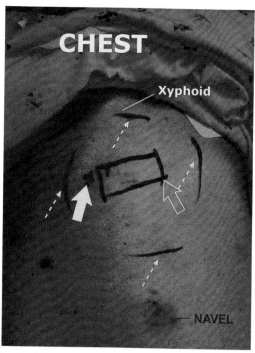

Fig. 1. Skin markings just before surgical preparation and draping. We like to mark the transducer orientation (*box, hollow white arrow*), the needle entry site (*black cross, solid white arrow*), and the estimated outline of the fenestrated drape (*dashed white arrows*). This strategy helps with patient safety and identification, helps the ancillary staff orient the room (ultrasound positioning, fluoroscopic C-arm position, and position of personnel) as well as the outline of the preparation or draping. The markings are universal and unmistakable.

infiltrated under the skin along the trajectory planned for the ablation probe using a 21-gauge needle. A small skin nick, large enough for the ablation probe to easily slide through, is made in the skin using an 11-blade scalpel. A sterile transducer cover should be placed on the ultrasound transducer along with the guide bracket (see **Fig. 2**). The target and the predetermined path are then identified. Depending on the ablation kit, a coaxial needle (see **Fig. 2**) or trocar may be placed first, through which the probe is subsequently placed. This strategy is believed to reduce tumor seeding of the tract, although ablation of the tract is believed to be the most effective method to prevent seeding.[9] The trocar or probe is placed into the target under direct visualization with ultrasound, using the guide bracket per standard biopsy technique (see **Fig. 2**). The probe can also be placed freehand with ultrasound visualization. If a trocar is in place, a biopsy can be performed and the needle exchanged for the

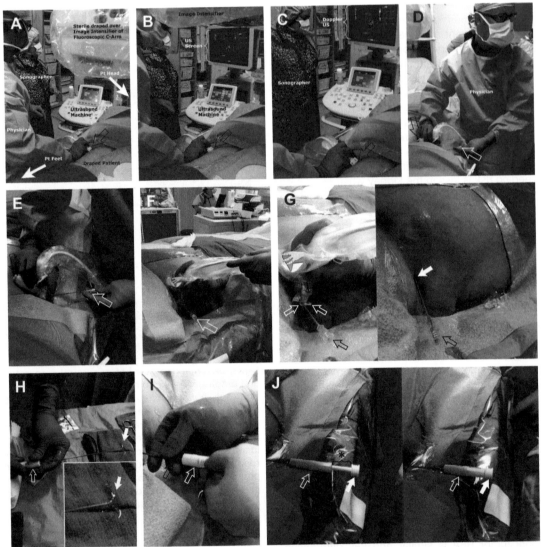

Fig. 2. (*A–C*) Combined ultrasound-guided and fluoroguided thermal ablation of 2 liver lesions. (*A*) Orientation of the operators to the patient with both ultrasound machine and operators to the right of the patient. The draped image intensifier of the fluoroscopic C-arm is raised to allow ample space for the operator to maneuver with the ultrasound transducer (*hollow black arrow*) as he looks at the ultrasound (US) machine screen. Once the operator identifies the target lesion(s) by gray-scale ultrasound (*B*), the operator switches to Doppler ultrasound (*C*) to iden-tify and orient himself with the hepatic vessels and choose a path with the least vasculature toward the target lesion(s). This process is a large part of the technical planning of the procedure. The room, operator, and patient orientation are predetermined before entering the room by the team to reduce room time and confusion around the patient. (*D–F*) Advancement of a coaxial ablation sheath (*hollow white arrow*) under real-time gray-scale ultra-sound guidance. The operator here is not advancing the sheath freehand but is using an ultrasound-transducer guide (hardware bracket) fixated to the ultrasound transducer (*hollow black arrow*). The photographs are obtained from different viewpoints. (*D*) In particular is facing the operator and between the patient (to the left) and the ultrasound machine to the right (*not shown*). (*G*) Before and after dismantling (disassembling) the ultrasound-transducer guide-bracket (*hollow white arrows*) from around the coaxial ablation sheath (*hollow black arrow*). The ultrasound transducer guide bracket (*hollow white arrows*) is designed to fall away from the sheath (*hollow black arrow*) without altering its position at the entry site (*solid white arrow*). (*H, with a magnified inset*) RFA probe (*hollow white arrow*) before it is inserted coaxially through the coaxial ablation sheath (which is now in the patient, see *D–H*). The operator is deploying the RFA tines (*solid white arrows*) to test the device before placing it into the patient. (*I*) The operator coaxially advances and screws secure the RFA probe (*hollow white arrow*) into the coaxial ablation sheath (*hollow black arrow*). (*J*) The operator is deploying the RFA tines in the liver lesion by pushing the plunger (*solid white arrows*) of the RFA probe (*hollow white arrows*). Notice the distance (*asterisk*) between plunger and main probe has disappeared on the second image. At this moment, the RFA probe is connected to the RFA machine to commence ablation (once the tines are confirmed to be in the target lesion by imaging).

ablation probe. Tip placement is dependent on the ablation device being used. After the needle tip is in the appropriate location within the tumor, it is exchanged for an ablation probe and the ablation is performed.

The most commonly used RFA systems are the LeVeen Needle Electrode (Boston Scientific, Natick, MA, USA), RITA Starburst RFA Probe (RITA, Mountain View, CA, USA), and the Radionics RFA Probe (Cool-Tip Radionics, Burlington, MA, USA).[4] These all are monopolar probes requiring a grounding pad on the patient's thigh. The LeVeen Needle probe has 10 tines, which deploy in a palm-tree–shaped array and come in various sizes chosen to correlate with tumor size (2.0, 3.0, 3.5, 4.0, and 5.0 cm). The tip of the LeVeen Needle should be placed just short of the center of the lesion because its tines open at the probe tip or slightly forward to the tip. The LeVeen Needle Electrode system has a unique impedance feedback mechanism.

The RITA Starburst RFA Probe deploys 7 to 9 tines in a starburst pattern, as the name suggests. Array diameters from 2 to 5 cm can be selected (7 tines for 2-cm to 3-cm lesions; 9 tines for 3-cm to 5-cm). The tip of the RITA probe should be placed at the superficial aspect of the tumor because its tines deploy forward and radially. The RITA probe infuses saline during the ablation to increase conductivity. It uses a 14-gauge trocar and monitors temperature in real time at the tip of each hook. Using a 100-W to 200-W RF generator, energy is applied for 10 to 15 minutes at a time. Larger lesions can take up to 60 minutes to treat and may require rotation or adjustment of the probe.[10] RFA is initiated and terminated either based on imaging characteristics or an automated system based on impedance.

The Radionics RFA probe is 17-gauge with 1 or 3 internally water-cooled needles in a cluster with a 200-W, 480-kHz RF generator. The single needle probe has 3 cm of exposed tip and can treat lesions up to 2 cm, whereas the clustered electrode can treat lesions up to 3 cm with a single placement. The Radionics ablation is guided by an automated, impedance-based algorithm. On average, 1800 mA of energy is applied, more for the clustered electrode and less for the single tine. Each ablation cycle lasts 8 to 12 minutes, with total procedure time of 12 to 15 minutes for single, small lesions. Larger lesions requiring multiple ablations require a proportionate amount of additional time. If a lesion is egg-shaped and percutaneously feasible, the probe is passed along the long axis with a subsequent multiple station approach. The probe should be deployed at the deepest end of the lesion and pulled back with overlap at the ablation sites.

Pulling the probe back requires retraction of the tines before position adjustment, with redeployment once in the desired location.

Familiarity with the ablation zone size for a given device is important. Sometimes multiple probes can be used, but one must be mindful that these probes used together have a synergistic effect and the end-ablation volume is generally greater than the sum of the normal ablation zone of each probe. Multiple probes should be placed 1 to 2 cm from each other and the boundary of the tumor and should be activated simultaneously. For a tumor adjacent to larger vessels, probes should be no more than 1 cm apart near the vessel and within 5 mm of the tumor boundary.

For more complicated lesions, several techniques have been developed that widen the spectrum of treatable lesions. Some lesions may require a laparoscopic or open surgical approach (explained further in the section on liver tumors), but most can be performed percutaneously. Hydrodissection involves injection of fluid to displace adjacent tissues, such as bowel, from the ablation zone, providing thermal and electrical insulation. Normal saline should not be used, because this can conduct the RF signals in a wider range; D5W (5% dextrose in water) is generally used. The same principle applies to creation of artificial ascites when treating hepatic dome lesions to prevent diaphragmatic injury. For renal lesions near the collecting system, pyeloperfusion (irrigating through a ureteral stent) creates a heat sink that protects the collecting system. Simple maneuvers such as repositioning the patient or using the probe itself to manipulate the position of the tumor can help to displace the lesion from adjacent structures as well.[7] At the end of the tumor ablation, the tract may be ablated to prevent seeding.

As with RFA, cryoablation should be performed per the device manufacturer's protocol. Endocare (Irvine, CA, USA) and Galil Medical (Wallingford, CT, USA) are the primary cryoprobe manufacturers. The systems are integrated with a computer monitoring system and can operate 7 to 8 probes simultaneously. The probes range in size from 1.5 to 8 mm. The Galil device is magnetic resonance (MR) compatible.[4] Cryoablation can be monitored with ultrasound but the ice-ball creates a highly echogenic mass, resulting in significant artifact and poor visualization of the posterior aspect of the ice-ball. Therefore, computed tomography (CT) and MR imaging are more commonly used to monitor cryoablation.[11] During cryoablation, care must be taken not to manipulate the probes while freezing, because this can cause ice-ball or organ cracking. Usually 1 or 2 thaw cycles are required for treatment with temperatures ranging from −120° to 40°C. The cryoprobe tip is placed just deep to the center of the lesion.[11]

POSTPROCEDURAL CARE AND FOLLOW-UP

Patients are closely monitored in the hospital overnight after ablation for observation and pain control. Immediate postprocedural ultrasonography is commonly nondiagnostic because of shadowing artifact. However, postprocedural ultrasonography may be helpful in documentation of capsular or subcapsular hematoma and serve as a baseline. On postoperative day 1, a repeat laboratory evaluation should be obtained, including complete blood count, comprehensive metabolic panel, and coagulation profile.

Postprocedural pain is common and can last from 2 to 5 days after the procedure. Some cases require narcotic oral pain medication or rarely patient-controlled analgesia. Cryoablation typically is less painful.[12] Soft tissue damage from probe passes, organ capsular damage, and abdominal wall or diaphragm damage contribute to worsened pain. Low-grade fever, malaise, and nausea occur in up to 40% of patients and are categorized as postablation syndrome, which usually starts about 48 hours after the procedure and can last up to 5 to 10 days. Treatment with nonsteroidal antiinflammatory drugs, acetaminophen, and antiemetics is appropriate.[7] Some institutions administer antibiotics for 5 to 7 days.

Most postablation patients are followed with a rigorous imaging regimen specific to their primary diagnosis. After the procedure baseline contrast-enhanced CT or MR imaging is performed at 24 hours to assess the extent of tumor treatment. Subsequently, patients are often followed with contrast-enhanced imaging at 1-month, 3-month, 6-month, and 12-month time points, with yearly follow-up thereafter to evaluate for recurrence. Contrast-enhanced ultrasound may also be used, per institution and operator preference. Diffusion-weighted MR imaging and fluorodeoxyglucose positron emission tomography imaging are also useful modalities for problem-solving cases in which there is an uncertain diagnosis of recurrence in the ablation bed. At the time of imaging follow-up, tumor markers and liver function or kidney function tests should be performed, if applicable.

LIVER TUMORS
Indications

Treatment indications for liver tumors vary depending on tumor type and location. Early-stage malignancies in the liver can be treated by partial liver resection, living or cadaveric liver transplantation, or one of the ablation modalities discussed herein. All options should be carefully considered for each patient. Surgical resection for HCC is indicated only for patients who have good functional reserve of the liver, normal bilirubin levels, a single and asymptomatic nodule, and no evidence of significant portal hypertension. Transplantation for HCC is limited by long wait lists, the requirement for decompensated liver disease, and solitary masses less than 5 cm or multiple masses, fewer than 3, and all less than 3 cm in size.[13] Cadaveric transplantation is limited by donors, whereas living donor transplantation is limited by donor-safety issues and its current lack of wide availability. Ablation is indicated when surgery is contraindicated and if the tumor and adjacent anatomy are not prohibitive (explained further later).

Liver tumors are classified as either primary (HCC) or secondary (metastatic disease). The treatment of primary liver tumors is the main indication of hepatic RFA. RFA may be performed in patients with unresectable HCC, as bridging therapy before transplantation, as a primary treatment of resectable HCC, or in patients with recurrent HCC after resection.[14] The patients treated with RFA for primary tumors include those with HCC superimposed on cirrhosis, nonsurgical candidates, disease confined to the liver, and disease that does not invade intrahepatic vasculature. Secondary tumors, or metastatic lesions, are less commonly treated with RFA but may be treated with success. The largest experience of RFA in secondary disease is in patients with colorectal cancer.[15] Patients with 1 to 5 asynchronous metastatic lesions that are 3 to 4 cm in maximal diameter may be treated with RFA. Larger lesions may be debulked with neoadjuvant chemotherapy before RFA. Ideally, no extrahepatic disease should be present.[5] Other secondary tumors that have been treated include patients with neuroendocrine, gastric, renal, melanoma, bronchogenic, uterine, ovarian, and breast metastases; however, full treatment options should be discussed with a multidisciplinary team on a case-by-case basis. Candidates for RFA treatment include patients with fewer than 4 to 5 lesions, no vascular invasion, and no extrahepatic dissemination.

Contraindications

The only true absolute contraindication for ablation is coagulopathy, with suggested thresholds as detailed earlier. Obstructive jaundice (bilirubin >3 mg/dL), neoplastic portal vein thrombosis, ascites, and hepatorenal failure are relative contraindications to ablation. Patients with pacemakers should be closely monitored during the procedure and have their device interrogated after the ablation.[16]

Tumor location near the hilum or gallbladder is not a contraindication, but care must be taken to avoid thermal injury to the biliary system and the possibility of iatrogenic cholecystitis. Adjacent vasculature is not a contraindication to ablation, because its heat-sink effect protects the vessel wall from damage. However, this same heat sump can result in adjacent residual tumor burden because of this characteristic. In addition, care must be taken to avoid needle puncture of large vessels. Ablation of lesions near the liver surface or at the hepatic dome should be avoided, because injury to the adjacent intestines can occur, with the large bowel being more sensitive to thermal injury than the small bowel or stomach. However, in experienced hands, repositioning of the patient or probe or the creation of artificial ascites can displace the intestines and allow for treatment. These types of lesions should be considered higher risk and require careful planning with a multidisciplinary team. Some of these tumors may be considered for intra-operative ablation (explained later).

Special Anatomic Considerations and Technique

In patients with HCC, the tumor must be nodular, focal, and relatively easily identified for targeting purposes. Diffuse infiltrating tumors are difficult to treat with RFA. Tumor size is important and should not exceed 3.5 to 4 cm, to obtain a 1-cm ablation margin. With metastatic lesions, patients with up to 5 asynchronous lesions less than 4 cm in size can be ablated.[4] A preablative ultrasound scan is necessary to assess interval tumor progression from previous imaging, sometimes excluding patients from RFA treatment. The examination also confirms the anatomy of adjacent organs and aids in determining an optimal access route. Access routes include intercostal, subcostal, and subxyphoid approaches.

General techniques for patient preparation and tumor access are detailed earlier. Local analgesia of the hepatic capsule (Glisson capsule) in addition to the skin and subcutaneous tissue is of utmost importance. An incision is made using an 11-blade scalpel, usually 3 mm deep. Coaxial needle access is obtained. If a midaxillary intercostal approach is used, the access needle should be passed cephalad to the ribs to avoid neurovascular injury below the ribs. Once access is obtained, the RFA probe is connected to the generator and advanced to the ablation site under ultrasound guidance. Details of probe technology and use are above and per the manufacturers' instructions. As described earlier,

patients with tumor near the surface or dome of the liver may require displacement of bowel. This goal may be achieved with proper patient positioning, adjustment of probe trajectory, or other percutaneous methods. Artificial ascites can be created with D5W to insulate structures such as the diaphragm or to displace the gallbladder or colon away from the ablation zone.[16]

Intra-operative Tumor Considerations

In addition to surface (subdiaphragmatic) lesions or those adjacent to other important structures, intra-operative tumor ablation may be used in certain conditions: preplanned ablation of a small lesion in a liver remnant during resection of a larger lesion to reduce resection size; underestimation of tumor size during preoperative evaluation or progression of disease between initial evaluation and operative date; and underestimation of degree of liver disease (cirrhosis), thereby changing the operative candidacy of the patient from a residual liver volume standpoint. As explained earlier, careful patient evaluation with review of cross-sectional imaging should be performed to evaluate tumor involvement. However, in some cases, there is progression of disease, requiring intra-operative tumor ablation.

The ablation can be performed through a laparoscope or by direct visualization during an open laparotomy (**Fig. 3**). The intra-operative approach has been performed in primary and secondary liver disease, with reported success.[17–19] Once the RFA probe is placed intra-operatively, the remainder of the technique is similar to the percutaneous approach. Radiologists performing intra-operative ablation must be cognizant of the orientation of organs and needles because they are different from what they are familiar with when performing percutaneous ablations. This situation can be seen in **Figs. 3** and **4**, in which the needle probe is passed subhepatically, close to the falciform ligament, with the liver raised by surgical retractors. Such an approach is impossible from a percutaneous standpoint. Also, the ultrasound images appear inverted where the hepatic veins and inferior vena cava (IVC) are seen in the deep end of the ultrasound image and the hepatic vein and portal vein bifurcations are seen superficially (see **Figs. 3** and **4**). In addition to the advantages of the various access approaches and potential short tract to the lesion, intra-operative ablation obviates tract ablation because the surgeon has direct access to the liver entry point (at the capsule) where electrocautery (Bovie) may be used to cauterize the tract and liver surface, reducing the risk of bleeding and tumor seeding (see **Fig. 4**).

384

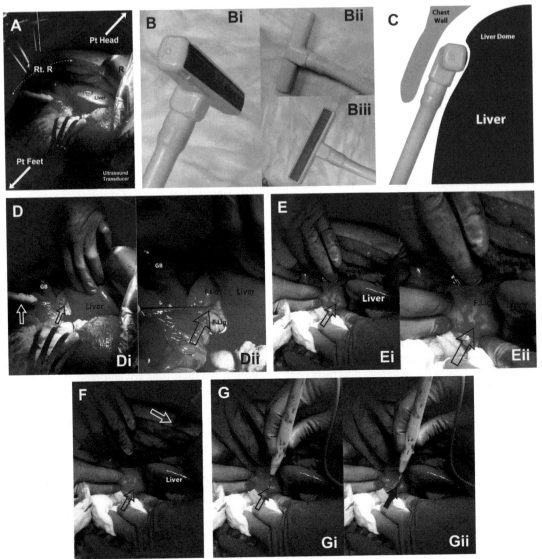

Fig. 3. Intra-operative tumor ablation in which the patient's liver cirrhosis was underestimated preoperatively. These photographic images belong to the same case (radiographic images) as **Fig. 4**. (*A*) Intra-operative photo-graph taken during a combined ultrasound-guided thermal ablation of a liver lesion showing the orientation of the patient and the right upper quadrant abdomen. The right subcostal margin (*dashed line with arrows*) is retracted by the right-sided subcostal retractor (Rt. R). On the other side of the abdomen is the left-sided subcos-tal retractor (Lt. R). The RFA probe (*hollow white arrow*) is seen entering the undersurface of the liver (difficult to achieve by percutaneous means) with its entry site (*hollow black arrow*) at the falciform ligament. Adjacent is the gallbladder (GB). (*B*) T-configured or hammerhead ultrasound transducer in multiple projections (*Bi–Biii*), which is typically used for intra-operative image-guided interventions such as biopsies and tumor ablations. It is config-ured this way because many of the planned elective intra-operative cases (biopsies or ablations) are high up in the liver dome (see *C*), which is safer to perform with open or laparoscopic surgery. This strategy applies not only to dome lesions but to all subcapsular diaphragmatic lesions. (*C*) Lateral photograph of the T-configured ultrasound transducer with a superimposed illustration showing how it is used (and why it is shaped) to visualize lesions that are high up in the liver just below the diaphragm. (*D*) Two intra-operative photographs taken after the left lobe of the liver (Liver) is raised to expose the undersurface of the liver. The RFA probe (*Di: hollow white arrow*) is seen entering the undersurface of the liver with its entry site (*hollow black arrow*) at the falciform liga-ment (*Dii*: F.Lig). Adjacent is the gallbladder (GB). (*E*) Two intra-operative photographs taken after the liver lesion has been ablated and with the left lobe of the liver (Liver) raised to expose the undersurface of the liver. The falciform ligament (*Eii*: F.Lig) is spread to expose the RFA probe entry site (*hollow black arrow*) so that the probe entry site does not touch any adjacent structures. (*F*) Next, a surgical cauterizing device (*hollow white arrow*) is applied to the RFA probe entry site (*hollow black arrow*) (also see *I*). (*G*) Two photographs (*Gi*: Early and *Gii*: Late) during the cauterization of the RFA probe access site at the falciform ligament. The purpose of this cauterization is for hemostasis and to prevent track seeding. As can be seen, the cauterized burn increases from early (*hollow black arrow*) to late (*solid black arrow*).

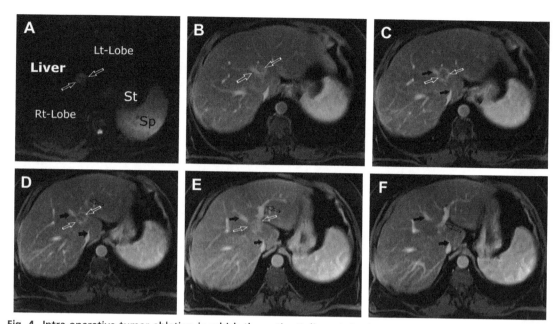

Fig. 4. Intra-operative tumor ablation in which the patient's liver cirrhosis was underestimated preoperatively. These photographic images belong to the same case as **Fig. 3.** (*A*) T2-weighted axial image showing a hyperintense lesion in a 53-year-old male patient with history of colon cancer. (*B–F*) T1-weighted contrast-enhanced axial images from cephalad (*B*) to caudad (*F*) showing a rim-enhancing lesion (*hollow white arrow*) situated between the middle hepatic vein (*solid black arrow*) and the left portal vein (*hollow black arrow*). (*G–I*) Gray-scale ultrasound images showing a rim-enhancing lesion (*hollow white arrow*) situated between the middle hepatic vein (*solid black arrow*) and the left portal vein (*hollow black arrow*). The images are upside down because the ultrasound probe is intra-abdominal and imaging is from the inferior margin of the liver. The left portal vein (*black hollow arrow*) is inferior (caudad) to the lesion (between *hollow white arrows* and centered by the *asterisk*) and the left hepatic vein (*solid black arrows*) is superior (cephalad) to the lesion as seen extending into the inferior vena cava (IVC) near the hepatic dome. (*J–L*) Gray-scale ultrasound images panning the ultrasound transducer from 1 side of the lesion to the other side after passing the RFA trocar needle (*solid white arrow* at needle tip) into the center of the lesion. Again seen is the left portal vein inferior (caudad) to the lesion (images are upside down because the ultrasound probe is intra-abdominal and imaging is from the inferior margin of the liver). (*M–P*) Gray-scale ultrasound images panning the ultrasound transducer from 1 side of the lesion to the other side after deploying the tines (*solid white arrows*) of the RFA probe coaxially through the trocar needle. Again seen is the left portal vein inferior (caudad) to the lesion (images are upside down because the ultrasound probe is intra-abdominal and imaging is from the inferior margin of the liver). (*Q*) Gray-scale ultrasound images during the RFA showing air/cavitation around the RFA probe tines. Notice the artifact (*brackets* and *bidirectional arrow*) seen from the RFA. Again seen is the left portal vein (LPV) inferior (caudad) to the lesion (images are upside down because the ultrasound probe is intra-abdominal and imaging is from the inferior margin of the liver). (*R*) Gray-scale ultrasound images during the RFA showing air/cavitation (between *solid white arrows*) around the RFA probe tines just cephalad to the left portal vein (LPV). (*S, T*) Contrast-enhanced CT images obtained 4 weeks after the ablation showing complete ablation of the lesion (between *hollow arrows*). (*U–W*) Contrast-enhanced CT sagittal reformats obtained 4 weeks after the ablation showing complete ablation of the lesion (*hollow arrows*). The ablated lesion/area is again seen situated between the confluence (Conf) of the middle (MHV) and left (LHV) hepatic veins and the left portal vein (LPV) proximally. (*X–AA*) Contrast-enhanced CT coronal reformats obtained 4 weeks after the ablation showing complete ablation of the lesion (*hollow arrows*). The ablated lesion/area is again seen situated between the confluence of the middle (MHV) and left (LHV) hepatic veins and the left portal vein (LPV) proximally just after the main portal vein (MPV) bifurcates into the right (RPV) and the left (LPV) portal vein.

Complications

Complications specific to hepatic tumor ablation include those involving the pleura/thoracic cavity, bowel perforation, abscess formation, liver failure, needle tract seeding, and cholecystitis. Mortality from thermal ablation ranges from 0.1% to 0.5%. Major complications occur in about 2.2% to 3.1% of cases, although rates as high as 7% have been reported.[20] Bleeding is usually self-limited; however, it is the most common

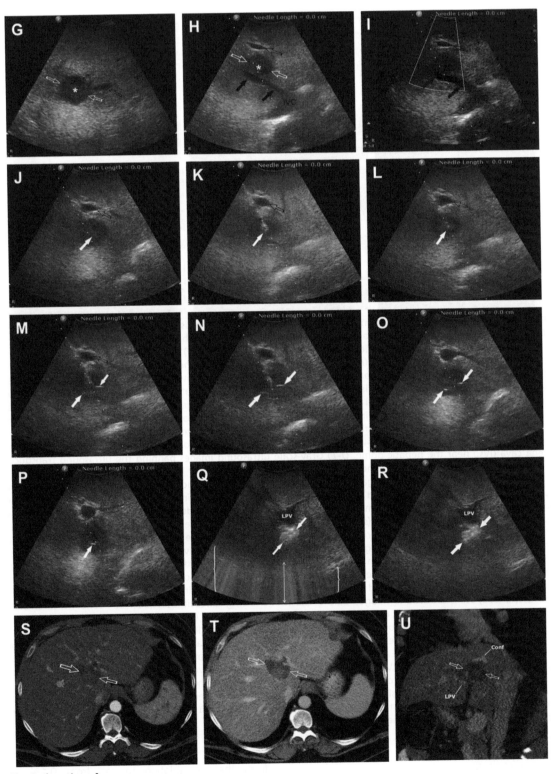

Fig. 4. (continued)

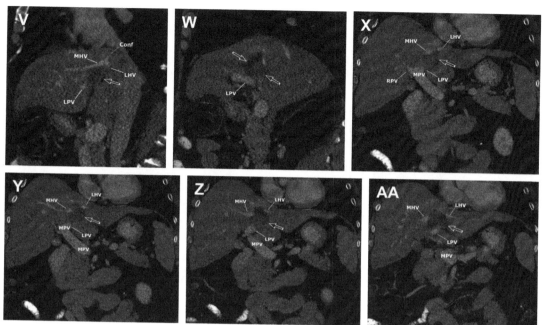

Fig. 4. (*continued*)

complication. Pneumothorax or hemothorax may present similarly to irritant peritonitis. A change in oxygen saturation in addition to chest pain should be evaluated with a chest radiograph. Supplemental oxygen and chest tube placement in addition to bleeding management may be required. Bowel perforation is usually delayed and occurs most frequently in the colon. A surgical consultation should be obtained and antibiotics administered as needed. Abscess formation may also be managed with antibiotics, in addition to percutaneous drainage, if applicable.

Tumor seeding of the ablation tract occurs in less than 0.5% of patients.[20] Ablation of the probe tract with RF should be performed if possible to reduce the chance of seeding, especially in lesions that require multiple punctures or subcapsular/peripheral tumors. Seeding can be managed with tract ablation, surgical resection, or palliation. Concern of tumor seeding should be reported to the liver transplant service because this may change transplantation candidacy.

Liver failure and cholecystitis should be managed with supportive therapy and appropriate medical and surgical consultation as necessary. Other less common complications include portal vein thrombosis, biloma, bile duct fistula or stricture, and grounding-pad–related skin burns. A rare complication of cryoablation is cryoshock, which is similar to tumor lysis syndrome. As the ice-ball melts, some reperfusion occurs and can cause some adverse events, including consumptive coagulopathy, thrombocytopenia, liver failure, renal failure, and rarely death.

Outcomes

Initial response rates of HCC to RFA are in the range of 85% to 95% (see **Fig. 4**; **Figs. 5** and **6**). Five randomized controlled trials have been performed comparing percutaneous ethanol injection (PEI) with RFA. Two of these trials reported a survival advantage with RFA, whereas 4 reported improved local tumor control with RFA. The most recent trial in 2011 showed 5-year survival of 68% in the PEI group and 70% in the RFA group, with a higher complication rate in the RFA group. In this trial, all tumors were solitary and less than 3 cm.[21] In the 2005 trial by Shiina and colleagues,[22] criteria were less strict and included patients with less than 3 tumors, all less than 3 cm in size. Four-year survival was 74% and 57% in the RFA and PEI groups, respectively. There was no difference in adverse events between groups in this trial. Interpreting these results, there is a good argument for using PEI on solitary tumors less than 3 cm, when considering cost is dramatically lower. However, more treatments are required, reflecting less robust local tumor control. The need for repeated treatments negatively affects quality of life in these patients, who are usually living out the last days of their lives. A 2007 study by Zhang and colleagues[23] suggests that there may be a therapeutic benefit to

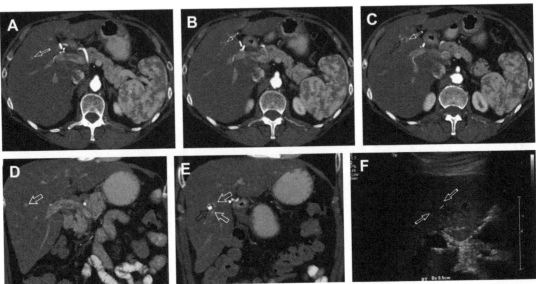

Fig. 5. Radiographic images of a percutaneous tumor ablation that belong to the same case as **Fig. 2**. (*A–C*) Three contrast-enhanced 5-mm slice axial CT images from cephalad (*A*) to caudad (*C*) of a middle-aged woman with history of HCC and is status post transcatheter chemoembolization. The patient has recurrence in 2 small lesions (*white hollow arrows*): 1 lesion (*B, C, hollow arrow*) at the periphery of the previously chemoembolized lesion with residual lipiodol within it (*hollow black arrow*). The second lesion is more cephalad (*A, hollow arrow*). (*D, E*) Two contrast-enhanced coronal reformats showing the 2 lesions (*white hollow arrows*): the first is the lesion (*E, hollow arrow*) at the periphery of the previously chemoembolized lesion with residual lipiodol within it (*hollow black arrow*) and the second lesion is more cephalad (*D, hollow arrow*). (*F, G*) Gray-scale images visualizing the lesion around the lipiodol (between *white hollow arrows*) being targeted with the needle tip of the ablation probe introducer (*solid white arrow*) in the center of the lesion. (*H*) Fluoroscopic image of the tip of the LeVeen ablation probe in the lesion that is adjacent to the lipiodol (*hollow black arrow*). The diamond tip (*solid white arrow*) extends beyond the trocar introducer (*hollow white arrow*). (*I*) Fluoroscopic image of the tip of the LeVeen ablation probe in the lesion that is adjacent to the lipiodol (*hollow black arrow*). The diamond tip has been removed, leaving the hollow trocar introducer (*hollow white arrow*). (*J*) Nonpulsatile bleeding was noted from the trocar introducer needle. The operator injected contrast to identify the nature of the vascular bleed. The fluoroscopic image shows that the bleeding is from a hepatic vein. In our opinion, this is not a significant injury from a bleeding standpoint. However, the hepatic vein may be a source of heat dissipation, limiting the effectiveness of RFA in reaching an effective thermal-therapeutic injury to the lesion. The operator proceeded with the ablation. Again noted is the trocar tip (*hollow white arrow*), which is in the hepatic vein and the lipiodol concentrate (*hollow black arrow*) is again noted. (*K*) Fluoroscopic image after coaxial deployment of the LeVeen ablation probe through the trocar introducer and into the lesion that is adjacent to the lipiodol (*hollow black arrow*). The tines (*hollow white arrows* on 2 of them) of the probe are visualized. (*L*) Gray-scale ultrasound image with the tines (*hollow white arrows*) of the ablation probe deployed in the lesion. (*M, N*) Two axial images of an intraprocedural Dyna-CT (rotational dynamic CT from the angiography suite without contrast). The tines of the ablation probe (*hollow arrows*) are seen deeper than the lipiodol concentrate (*hollow black arrows*). This is where the lesion is situated (see *B* and *C*). The shaft (*solid white arrows*) of the probe is seen traversing the abdominal wall and liver (*solid white arrow*). (*O*) Gray-scale ultrasound image after the ablation of the lesion. The probe (*solid white arrows*) is still situated in the lesion. Cavitation is seen around the lesion (between *hollow arrows*). (*P*) Fluoroscopic image after redeployment of the probe after it has been repositioned with an overlap with the previous ablation lesion. Again seen are the tines (*hollow white arrows*). (*Q*) Fluoroscopic image after the second overlapping ablation. Under ultrasound and fluoroscopic guidance, the ablation probe is pulled gradually to ablate the transhepatic tract as the tines are retracted (*white hollow arrow*). (US-T: ultrasound transducer). (*R, S*) Gray-scale ultrasound images after redeployment of the probe into the more cephalad lesion. The tines (*hollow white arrows*) of the ablation probe deployed in the new lesion. (*T, U*) Fluoroscopic image after repositioning the ablation probe. Initially, the inner trocar needle has been removed (*T*), leaving the introducer trocar (*T, solid white arrow*) and the ablation probe has been replaced with its tines (*hollow white arrows*) deployed in the second lesion. (*V, W*) Contrast-enhanced axial CT images 4 weeks after the ablation showing the ablation area, which overlaps and encompasses the cephalad lesion (*V, hollow white arrow*) and the lesion (*W, hollow white arrow*) adjacent to the lipiodol spot. (*X*) Contrast-enhanced coronal reformats before and after (4 weeks after) the ablation, again showing the ablation area, which involves the area where the lesion was noted (*hollow white arrows*).

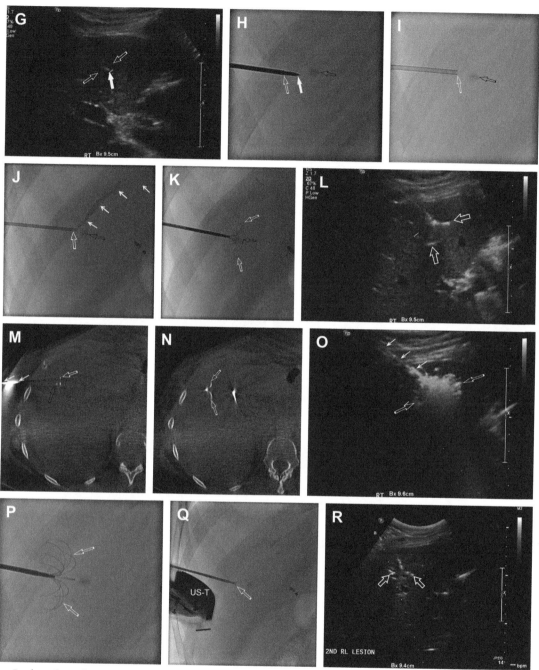

Fig. 5. (*continued*)

combination PEI/RFA in tumors that are 3.1 to 5.0 cm. Combination therapy also decreased local recurrence.

Comparing RFA with surgical resection, 1 study shows no difference in survival when a solitary sub–5-cm tumor is present. However, a study published by Huang and colleagues[24] in 2010 indicates better recurrence and survival rates in

patients after surgical resection. The 1-year, 2-year, 3-year, 4-year, and 5-year overall survival rates for the RFA group and the surgical resection group were 86.96%, 76.52%, 69.57%, 66.09%, 54.78% and 98.26%, 96.52%, 92.17%, 82.60%, 75.65%, respectively. Vivarelli and colleagues[25] reported 1-year and 3-year survival rates of 79% and 50% versus 60% and 20% with surgical

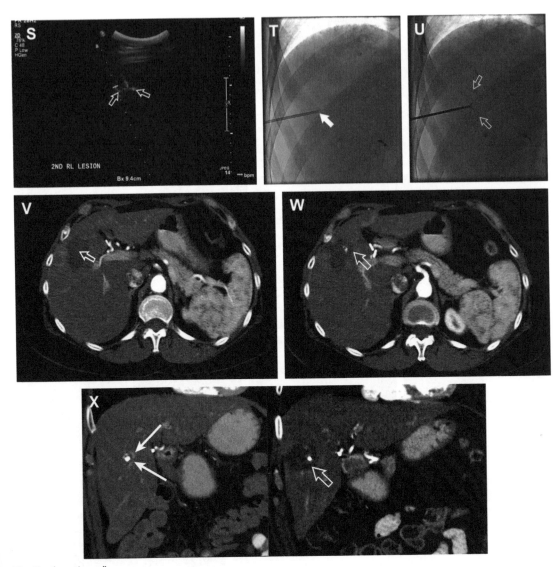

Fig. 5. *(continued)*

resection and RFA, respectively. These studies support the continued use of surgery as first-line therapy until RFA has been further studied.

Outcomes for RFA in colorectal metastatic disease seem to be comparable with surgery. Local control in the short-term seems to be as high as 82% to 90%, especially in patients with smaller tumors (<3 cm) and fewer than 5 lesions. However, these patients often present with asynchronous lesions within the first year. Five-year survival ranges from 14% to 55%.[26] Breast cancer metastases are the next most commonly treated secondary lesions using RFA. Surgical resection of breast cancer metastases in the liver has proved useful and results in up to 21% to 61% survival at 5 years.[27] Data are sparse in regards to RFA for

other metastatic lesions. Long-term data after cryotherapy are also limited. Studies have shown initially symptomatic relief after ablation of neuroendocrine tumors deemed to be unresectable. Initial success ranges from 60% to 85%, with recurrence rates from 3% to 53%. Studies in the surgical literature show no survival benefit of cryoablation when compared with standard surgical treatment of liver metastases.[5]

RENAL TUMORS
Indications

Current indications for renal tumor ablation are not well defined because of lack of clinical trials and definitive research but include small, 3-cm to

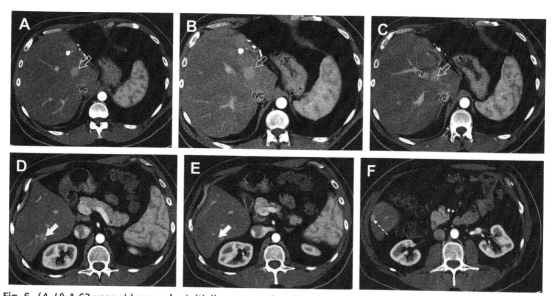

Fig. 6. (*A–H*) A 63-year-old man who initially presented with a ruptured left hepatic lobe HCC and is status post left lobectomy and chemoembolization of the right hepatic lobe (3 segmental chemoembolizations). He now presents with recurrent lesions. (*A–H*) Contrast-enhanced axial images from cephalad (*A*) to caudad (*H*). The images show 3 lesions, the largest of which (*hollow white arrow*) is situated immediately above the right portal vein (PV). The second lesion (*solid white arrow*) is capsular, with a deeper subcapsular component near Morison's pouch. The third lesion (*dashed white arrow*) is subcapsular near the inferior border of the liver. (*I–K*) Three contrast-enhanced coronal reformats from anterior (*I*) to posterior (*K*). The images again show the 3 lesions, the largest of which (*hollow white arrow*) is situated immediately above the right portal vein (PV). The second lesion (*dashed white arrow*) is subcapsular near the inferior border of the liver. The third lesion (*solid white arrow*) is capsular, with a deeper subcapsular component near Morison's pouch. (*L*) Gray-scale ultrasound image of the lesion (*hollow white arrow*) at Morison's pouch (correlate with the lesion by CT in *D–E* and *K*) adjacent to the right kidney (*K*). (*M, N*) Gray-scale ultrasound image of the lesion at Morison's pouch (correlate with the lesion by CT in *D, E, K*) as the RFA probe (*hollow white arrow*) is advanced into the lesion. (*O*) Gray-scale ultrasound image of the lesion at Morison's pouch (correlate with the lesion by CT in *D, E, K*) after RFA showing cavitation (between *hollow white arrows*) within the lesion. (*P*) Gray-scale ultrasound image of the subcapsular lesion (between *dashed white arrows*) at the lowermost margin of the liver (correlate with the lesion by CT in *F–H, J*). (*Q, R*) Gray-scale ultrasound image of the subcapsular lesion (correlate with the lesion by CT in *F–H, J*) as the RFA probe (*dashed white arrow*) is advanced into the lesion. (*S–U*) Noncontrast axial CT images of the subcapsular lesion (correlate with the lesion by CT in *F–H, J*) after the RFA probe (*hollow white arrow*) has been advanced and deployed in the lesion. The dashed white arrow (*U*) highlights the lack of distance of the large bowel to the target lesion/tines of the ablation probe. (*V–X*) Noncontrast axial CT images of the subcapsular lesion (correlate with the lesion by CT in *F–H, J*) after hydrodissection (injection of sterile water) using a needle (*hollow white arrow*) that has been placed adjacent to the RFA probe with its tines (*solid white arrow*) deployed. The *dashed white arrow* highlights the increasing distance (distraction) between the large bowel to the target lesion/tines of the ablation probe (compare distances with *S–U*). The cause of this successful distraction is the formation of a water-ball (*asterisk*), which has displaced the large bowel medially. (*Y*) Two coronal reformats of the noncontrast axial CT images of the subcapsular lesion (correlate with the lesion by CT in *F–H, J*) before (*left image*) and after (*right image*) hydrodissection (injection of sterile water) using a needle. The *dashed white arrow* on the *left image* (before hydrodissection) highlights the lack of distance between the large bowel and the ablation probe. The *bidirectional arrow* in the *right image* shows the successful distraction between the large bowel and the target lesion/tines of the ablation probe. (*Z*) Gray-scale ultrasound image of the largest lesion (*hollow white arrow*), which is situated just above the right portal vein (correlate with the lesion by CT in *A–C* and *I*). (*AA*) Gray-scale ultrasound image of the central lesion (correlate with the lesion by CT in *A–C* and *I*) after the RFA probe (*hollow white arrow*) has been advanced into the lesion. (*BB–EE*) Noncontrast axial CT images from cephalad (*BB*) to caudad (*EE*) of the central lesion (correlate with the lesion by CT in *A–C, I*) after the tines (*hollow white arrow*) of the RFA probe have been deployed. The *asterisks* mark the right portal vein, which is the continuation of the main portal vein (patient is status post left lobectomy). The tines are close to the central portal vein (*asterisks*). (*FF–OO*) Contrast-enhanced axial CT images from cephalad (*FF*) to caudad (*OO*) 1 month after RFA. The images show the complete ablation of the 3 lesions (*hollow black arrows*) that were seen enhancing in *A–H*.

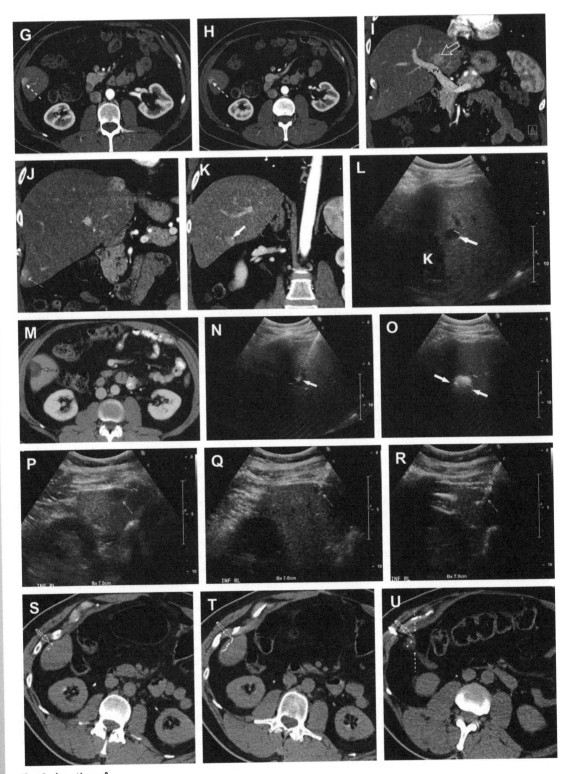

Fig. 6. (*continued*)

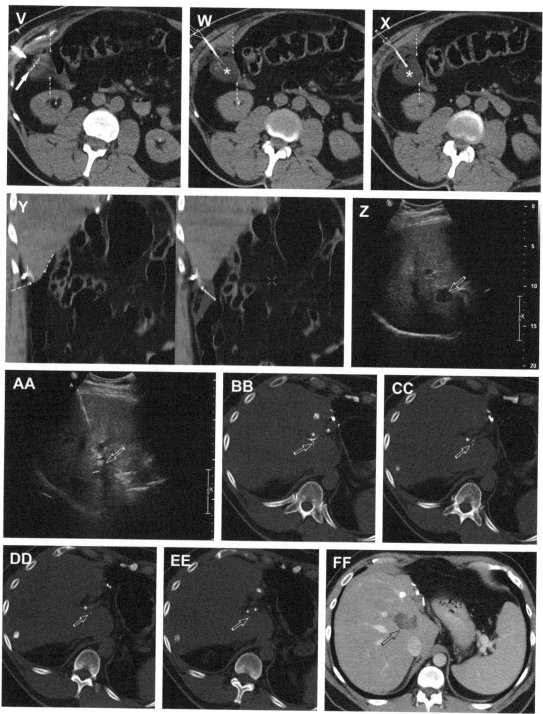

Fig. 6. (*continued*)

4-cm solid renal cell carcinoma (RCC) lesions that are confined to the kidney or renal arteriovenous malformations not amenable to endovascular treatment. Patients with poor renal function may be good candidates because these local therapies can help preserve remaining renal function. This factor becomes important in patients with diseases such as Von-Hippel-Lindau, who likely

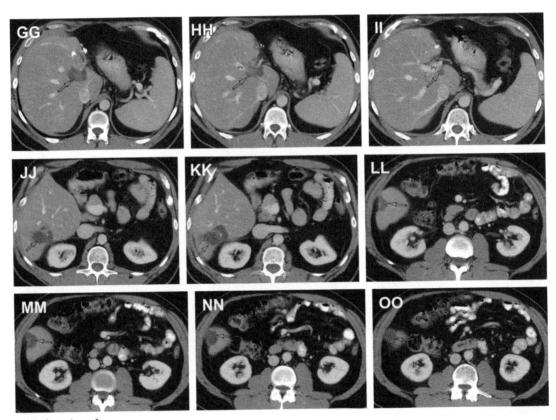

Fig. 6. (*continued*)

require multiple interventions over the course of their lifetime.[28] Patients such as these, who develop multifocal tumors, can benefit from ablation procedures that delay need for nephrectomies and dialysis. Patients with RCC in solitary, native kidneys or transplanted kidneys are ablative candidates. In addition, patients who are not surgical candidates for tumor resection, based on comorbid conditions, may be able to undergo less invasive ablations under conscious sedation. RFA can also be used palliatively to treat intractable hematuria secondary to tumor. Ablation is especially useful in treating patients with recurrence after nephrectomy or patients who would otherwise require multiple surgeries. When considering size, it has been suggested that only renal tumors less than 4 cm should be treated with RFA.[28,29]

Contraindications

As with other ablation procedures, uncorrectable coagulopathy is the only real absolute contraindication. Renal ablation should be performed as an elective treatment unless hematuria is the cause of instability. Septic patients should ideally be stabilized before ablative treatment.

Tumor ablation is not recommended in patients with extension of the tumor into the venous system, distant metastases, lymphatic involvement, and extension into adjacent organs. In addition, lesions that are anteromedially located and those adjacent to the ureteropelvic junction (UPJ) or proximal ureter have a higher risk of causing UPJ or ureteric injury and are therefore not treated with ablation. Patients with anteriorly located renal tumors are commonly better candidates for laparoscopic ablation and should be evaluated as such.

Special Anatomic Considerations and Technique

Exophytic masses of the kidney are easier to ablate because they are surrounded by fat, which insulates the ablation and allows for increased temperatures and prolonged times at those temperatures. Masses near the renal hilum are more difficult to treat, not only because of the proximity of the collecting system and large vessels, which are prone to injury, but also because of the heat-sink effect of these hilar structures, increasing the risk of incomplete tumor ablation.[30]

As with other tumors, preoperative trajectory planning using cross-sectional imaging is imperative to ensure no vital structures are traversed during probe placement. Special techniques can be used to protect or displace vital structures from the ablation zone. As described earlier, hydrodissection with instillation of sterile water or D5W can help displace and insulate structures. Insertion and inflation of a balloon can be used for displacement as well. Instillation of cooled or warmed solution (for RFA and cryoablation, respectively) through the collecting system via retrograde or antegrade ureteral stent can help protect the collecting system. Retrograde pyeloperfusion has been shown to allow complete tumor ablation of RCC within 1.5 cm (mean = 7 mm) of the collecting system. In addition, real-time temperature monitoring can aid in completion of tumor treatment. Access to the tumor should be attempted without crossing the pleural space, but a transthoracic approach with intentional pneumothorax creation has been reported for access to superior pole lesions.[16]

CT is the most common modality used for monitoring cryoablation, although ultrasonography may be used for intraprocedural monitoring in some cases. Biopsy can be performed immediately before the ablation; however, its usefulness is controversial because most small solid tumors in the kidney represent RCC. Biopsy may be valuable if there is concern that the lesion represents lymphoma or metastatic disease.

Complications

Complications in renal tumor ablation may include bleeding, pleural/thoracic cavity injury, bowel perforation, abscess formation, and needle tract tumor seeding as in hepatic tumor ablation, and should be managed similarly. Specific complications related to renal tumor ablation include retroperitoneal hemorrhage, hematuria, and urinary tract injury. Retroperitoneal hemorrhage may present as persistent severe back pain with or without hypotension. Patients should be evaluated with CT imaging of the abdomen and pelvis. Management includes fluid resuscitation, blood transfusion, and embolization or surgical treatment as needed. Hematuria and urinary tract injury also may necessitate intervention either percutaneously or surgically.

Outcomes

RCC accounts for most renal tumors ablated. For all tumor sizes and series, technical success for complete tumor ablation has ranged from 79% to 100%. More recent series with sub–4-cm tumors report success rates greater than 90%. Recurrence rates are around 5.3% at 2 years.[16,28,29,31] Ferakis and colleagues[31] showed a tumor control rate of 92% and 89% at 3 and 5 years, respectively. This rate is comparable with nephron-sparing surgical techniques. RFA in patients with a solitary kidney showed decreases in creatinine clearance by 16% on average, comparable with surgical therapies.[32]

Littrup and colleagues[33] showed an 8.3% recurrence or failure rate using cryoablation for solid renal tumors (most were RCC, but other tumor types were included). Matin and colleagues[34] examined 616 cases of ablation, RFA, and cryoablation. The investigators reported residual or recurrent disease in 3.9% of cryoablations and 13.4% of RFA cases. Most of these treatment failures were discovered within the first 3 months and successfully treated thereafter, resulting in a 2-year survival of 82.5% for those individuals with recurrent or residual disease. Overall, in patients with localized, unilateral renal tumors, the 2-year survival was 97.4%.

Johnson and coworkers examined complications of renal tumor ablation and found that major complications occurred in 1.8% of cases, death in 0.4%, and minor complications (mostly pain or paresthesia at probe insertion site) in 9.2% of cases.[35] Postprocedural care and follow-up are generally similar to liver ablation care as described earlier, with pain control, overnight observation, and contrast-enhanced imaging follow-up at 1, 3, 6, and 12 months and yearly thereafter.

ADRENAL AND OTHER TUMORS

RFA has been studied as a treatment option for benign (hormonally active), malignant, and metastatic tumors in the adrenal glands. However, CT-guided cryoablation is used by most institutions and operators, and therefore discussion in this article is limited. Indications are similar to other ablative procedures and include tumors near 3 cm in size in patients who are not appropriate surgical candidates.[36,37] Uncorrected coagulopathy is the main contraindication. Treatment of adrenal lesions requires careful planning because the liver, IVC, and aorta may be close to one another. The adrenal gland can be ablated via an anterior, lateral, or posterior approach. When the patient is placed prone, the adrenal glands are closer in position to the aorta and bowel. Again, the change in relationships of vital structures has to be carefully considered because there is an increased heat-sink effect in this position.

Adrenal lesions are more easily approached with CT guidance, but can be ablated using ultrasonography. It may be necessary to traverse the liver, kidney, or even spleen to ablate an adrenal lesion. Ablation can be performed safely, with care and attention to cauterization or embolization of the probe tract on its removal. Pheochromocytomas can be percutaneously ablated; however, hypertensive crisis from catecholamine release can be precipitated by the procedure. Standard prophylaxis must be undertaken preoperatively with initial α-adrenergic blockade and subsequent β-adrenergic blockade if needed. Definitive studies regarding long-term efficacy of adrenal tumor ablation are lacking and are a focus of future research.[36,37]

The breast, as a superficial organ, offers a prime opportunity for ablative tumor therapies using ultrasound guidance.[38] In addition, the fact that most breast tumors are surrounded by fat can allow for better ablation efficiency. Difficulty occurs with tumors close to the skin and chest wall, which increases the risk of complication.[39] Many radiologists have extensive experience in using ultrasound guidance for breast biopsy, and the technique for probe placement for ablation is nearly identical.

SUMMARY

Percutaneous tumor ablative therapies using ultrasound guidance have shown efficacy in local tumor control in a variety of organs and tumor types. Tumor ablation can be repeated multiple times and more easily than repeated surgery as necessary, and generally no bridges are burned. Surgery can be performed after an ablation if needed without added complication from the ablation procedure itself. Percutaneous ablation leaves smaller scars, providing a better cosmetic outcome than an open surgical procedure. As a complementary therapy, ablation can be used in conjunction with surgery, chemotherapy, or radiation.

The applicability of tumor ablation will continue to expand as we continue to study these modalities, with the goal of offering patients the most minimally invasive and curative therapies. Advancing technologies including probe design will continue to improve ablation profiles. The breast, prostate, and other organs have been studied for potential targets of ablative therapies. New technologies are constantly being developed and will expand the treatment possibilities for these minimally invasive techniques. Percutaneous and intra-operative ablation procedures have the potential to offer curative, minimally invasive treatment to patients who are unable to undergo surgical resection for local tumor control. To this end, randomized controlled trials are necessary to evaluate the efficacy of these modalities in tumor treatment to provide patients with the best treatment possible, offering the lowest morbidity and highest success rate.

REFERENCES

1. Clark TW. Chemical ablation of liver cancer. Tech Vasc Interv Radiol 2007;10:58–63.
2. Lencioni R, Crocetti L. Radiofrequency ablation of liver cancer. Tech Vasc Interv Radiol 2007;10:38–46.
3. Ahmed M, Brace CL, Lee FT, et al. Principles of and advances in percutaneous ablation. Radiology 2011; 258:351–69.
4. Dogra VS, Saad WE. Ultrasound-guided procedures. 1st edition. New York: Thieme; 2008.
5. Mauro MA, Murphy K, Thomson K, et al. Image-guided interventions: expert radiology series. 1st edition. Philadelphia: Saunders; 2008.
6. Garrean S, Hering J, Helton WS, et al. A primer on transarterial, chemical, and thermal ablative therapies for hepatic tumors. Am J Surg 2007;194:79–88.
7. Webb H, Lubner MG, Hinshaw JL. Thermal ablation. Semin Roentgenol 2011;46:133–41.
8. Hanna NN. Radiofrequency ablation of primary and metastatic hepatic malignancies. Clin Colorectal Cancer 2004;4(2):92–100.
9. Friedman M, Mikityansky I, Kam A, et al. Radiofrequency ablation of cancer. Cardiovasc Intervent Radiol 2004;27(5):427–34.
10. Ni Y, Mulier S, Miao Y, et al. A review of the general aspects of radiofrequency ablation. Abdom Imaging 2005;30:381–400.
11. Hinshaw JL, Lee FT. Cryoablation for liver cancer. Tech Vasc Interv Radiol 2007;10:47–57.
12. Sabel MS, Kaufman CS, Whitworth P, et al. Cryoablation of early-stage breast cancer: work-in-progress report of a multi-institutional trial. Ann Surg Oncol 2004;11(5):542–9.
13. Ng K. Radiofrequency ablation for malignant liver tumor. Surg Oncol 2005;14:41–52.
14. Lee WY, Lai EC. The current role of radiofrequency ablation in the management of hepatocellular carcinoma: a systematic review. Ann Surg 2009;249:20–5.
15. McKay A, Dixon E, Taylor M. Current role of radiofrequency ablation for the treatment of colorectal liver metastases. Br J Surg 2006;93:1192–201.
16. Krehbiel K, Ahmad A, Leyendécker J, et al. Thermal ablation: update and technique at a high-volume institution. Abdom Imaging 2008;33:695–706.
17. Kang CM, Lee KH, Kim KM, et al. "Dual-scopic" intra-operative radiofrequency ablation for the treatment of a hepatic metastatic tumor located beneath the diaphragm. Surg Laparosc Endosc Percutan Tech 2008;18:202–6.

18. Hammill CW, Billingsley KG, Cassera MA, et al. Outcome after laparoscopic radiofrequency ablation of technically resectable colorectal liver metastases. Ann Surg Oncol 2011;18:1947–54.

19. Hildebrand P, Kleemann M, Roblick U, et al. Laparoscopic radiofrequency ablation of unresectable hepatic malignancies: indication, limitation, and results. Hepatogastroenterology 2007;54:2069–72.

20. Decadt B, Siriwardena AK. Radiofrequency ablation of liver tumours: systematic review. Lancet Oncol 2004;5(9):550–60.

21. Giorgio A, Di Sarno A, De Stefano G, et al. Percutaneous radiofrequency ablation of hepatocellular carcinoma compared to percutaneous ethanol injection in treatment of cirrhotic patients: an Italian randomized controlled trial. Anticancer Res 2011;31(6):2291–5.

22. Shiina S, Teratani T, Obi S, et al. A randomized controlled trial of radiofrequency ablation with ethanol injection for small hepatocellular carcinoma. Gastroenterology 2005;129(1):122–30.

23. Zhang YJ, Liang HH, Chen MS, et al. Hepatocellular carcinoma treated with radiofrequency ablation with or without ethanol injection: a prospective randomized trial. Radiology 2007;244:599–607.

24. Huang J, Yan L, Cheng Z, et al. A randomized trial comparing radiofrequency ablation and surgical resection for HCC conforming to the Milan criteria. Ann Surg 2010;252(6):903–12.

25. Vivarelli M, Guglielmi A, Ruzzenente A, et al. Surgical resection versus percutaneous radiofrequency ablation in the treatment of hepatocellular carcinoma on cirrhotic liver. Ann Surg 2004;240(1):102–7.

26. Wong SL, Mangu PB, Choti MA, et al. American Society of Clinical Oncology 2009 clinical evidence review on radiofrequency ablation of hepatic metastases from colorectal cancer. J Clin Oncol 2009;28: 493–508.

27. Bergenfeldt M, Jensen BV, Skjoldbye B, et al. Liver resection and local ablation of breast cancer liver metastases–a systematic review. Eur J Surg Oncol 2011;37:549–57.

28. Stone MJ, Venkatesan AM, Locklin J, et al. Radiofrequency ablation of renal tumors. Tech Vasc Interv Radiol 2007;10:132–9.

29. Chiou S, Liu J, Needleman L. Current status of sonographically guided radiofrequency ablation techniques. J Ultrasound Med 2007;26:487–99.

30. Schiller JD, Gervais DA, Mueller PR. Radiofrequency ablation of renal cell carcinoma. Abdom Imaging 2005;30:442–50.

31. Ferakis N, Bouropoulos C, Granitsas T, et al. Long-term results after computed-tomography-guided percutaneous radiofrequency ablation for small renal tumors. J Endourol 2010;24(12):1909–13.

32. Syvanthong C, Wile GE, Zagoria RJ. Effect of radiofrequency ablation of renal tumors on renal function in patients with a solitary kidney. AJR Am J Roentgenol 2007;188(6):1619–21.

33. Littrup PJ, Ahmed A, Aoun HD, et al. CT-guided percutaneous cryotherapy of renal masses. J Vasc Interv Radiol 2007;18(3):383–92.

34. Matin SF, Ahrar K, Cadeddu JA, et al. Residual and recurrent disease following renal energy ablative therapy: a multi-institutional study. J Urol 2006; 176(5):1973–7.

35. Johnson DB, Solomon SB, Su LM, et al. Defining the complications of cryoablation and radio frequency ablation of small renal tumors: a multi-institutional review. J Urol 2004;172(3):874–7.

36. Venkatesan AM, Locklin J, Dupuy DE, et al. Percutaneous ablation of adrenal tumors. Tech Vasc Interv Radiol 2010;13:89–99.

37. Beland MD, Mayo-Smith WW. Ablation of adrenal neoplasms. Abdom Imaging 2008;34:588–92.

38. Oura S, Tamaki T, Hirai I, et al. Radiofrequency ablation therapy in patients with breast cancers two centimeters or less in size. Breast Cancer 2007; 14(1):48–54.

39. Manenti G, Bolacchi F, Perretta T, et al. Small breast cancers: in vivo percutaneous US-guided radiofrequency ablation with dedicated cool-tip radiofrequency system. Radiology 2009;251(2):339–46.

Percutaneous Transhepatic Biliary Drainage

Matthew R. Gossage, MD[a],*, Robert F. Short, MD, PhD[b],
Wael E. Saad, MBBCh, FSIR[c]

KEYWORDS

- Percutaneous transhepatic biliary drainage • Transhepatic biliary access
- Percutaneous transhepatic cholangiography • Biliary abnormalities

KEY POINTS

- Ultrasound can play an important role in transhepatic biliary access.
- There are no absolute contraindications but relative contraindications relate to uncorrected coagulopathy.
- Review of available imaging can be useful in planning the procedure.
- Postprocedurally, the patient's pain, laboratory values, and vital signs should be closely monitored.

INTRODUCTION

Percutaneous transhepatic cholangiography (PTC) is an effective procedure to diagnose and treat a variety of biliary abnormalities. The operator may elect for a right-sided or left-sided approach for PTC, or both. Generally, right-sided interventions are strictly performed under fluoroscopy. For a left-sided approach, ultrasound (US) plays an important role in visualization of the left hepatic lobe biliary ducts and vascular structures. US-guided targeting of biliary ducts under direct visualization allows more efficient PTC with or without percutaneous biliary drainage (PBD) placement and helps avoid vascular injury. This article focuses primarily on US-guided left-sided bile duct access.

INDICATIONS

PTC in general can be useful for both diagnostic and therapeutic purposes, with indications ranging from elective to emergent depending on the clinical scenario.

Diagnostic (PTC)

- Image cholangitis, obstructive biliary stones, or other inflammatory and neoplastic processes.
- Demonstrate postsurgical anatomy and/or a bile leak.
- Provide specific anatomic detail as to the level of the obstruction or abnormality.
- Biopsy of tumor.

Therapeutic

- Decompression of the dilated biliary tree
  - Biliary sepsis (emergent)
  - Pruritus
- Diversion of a bile leak
- Interventions
  - Stent placement across a stricture
  - Stone extraction.

PTC Versus Endoscopic Retrograde Cholangiopancreatography

In many instances, endoscopic retrograde cholangiopancreatography (ERCP) can be performed

[a] Department of Radiology and Medical Imaging, University of Virginia, 1215 Lee Street, PO Box 800170, Charlottesville, VA 22908, USA; [b] Department of Radiology, University of Pittsburgh Medical Center, Pittsburgh, PA, USA; [c] Division of Vascular Interventional Radiology, Department of Radiology and Imaging Sciences, University of Virginia Health System, Charlottesville, VA, USA
* Corresponding author.
E-mail address: MRG8P@hscmail.mcc.virginia.edu

Ultrasound Clin 7 (2012) 399–411
doi:10.1016/j.cult.2012.03.008
1556-858X/12/$ – see front matter © 2012 Elsevier Inc. All rights reserved.

more easily and should be considered as first line. The decision whether to perform PTC or ERCP is multifactorial; however, often cases arise where gastrointestinal access is limited (eg, gastric outlet obstruction, high intrahepatic obstructions, and postoperative anatomy), in which case PTC/PBD offers advantage over ERCP.

Right Versus Left PTC

The decision to perform left-sided PTC, alone or in conjunction with right-sided PTC, depends on operator preference and clinical scenario.

- For *asymmetric liver function* (atrophy, portal vein abnormalities), more benefit will be derived from drainage of the better functioning lobe.
- In cases of *segmental isolation* of right-sided ducts, a left-sided PDB may be provide better drainage.
- If there is *inadequate drainage* from a single access, eg, the left ducts remain dilated despite right PBD, bilateral drainage is required.

Right side
- Advantages:
  - Favorable anatomy for subsequent intervention
  - Larger drainage catchment
  - Less radiation exposure to operator during placement and subsequent PBD changes.
- Disadvantage:
  - More painful for patient.

Left side
- Advantages:
  - Less painful: avoid intercostal nerves
  - Less morbidity: avoid blood vessels
  - Less leakage with ascites (position)
  - More easily accessed and cared for by the patient.
  - Less likely for drain to fall out (better patient care).
- Disadvantages:
  - Difficult or impossible in cases of atrophic or a high-riding left hepatic lobe.
  - More likely to access a central duct instead of a preferred peripheral approach.

CONTRAINDICATIONS

There are no absolute contraindications, but relative contraindications relate to uncorrected coagulopathy and large-volume ascites.

- Uncorrected coagualopathy

- International normalized ratio (INR): >1.4
- Platelets: <50,000 to 70,000
- Partial thromboplastin time (PTT): >50 seconds. The clinician must take efforts to correct the coagulopathy, and must weigh this factor against the degree of clinical urgency to determine relative versus absolute contraindications.
- Large-volume ascites
  - Relative contraindication: increased risk for peritonitis, technical difficulty, and bleeding.
  - Addressed with periprocedural paracentesis.

RISKS

The overall major complication rate for PTC is on the order of 2% to 3% (with 21-gauge or smaller needles).

The primary risks related to PTC are

- Hemorrhage (less with left vs right)
- Infection
  - Biliary sepsis (life-threatening)
  - Cholangitis, abscess formation
- Pneumothorax (rare on left).

Bleeding is most often transient; however, in rare cases, can result in the need for blood transfusion, hepatic arterial embolization, or surgery. Addition of the PBD placement aspect increases procedure risk slightly, with a reported intraprocedural death rate of 1.7%. Risk depends on the patient's clinical scenario, with malignancy, cholangitis, and coagulopathy engendering increased risk.

PLANNING
Imaging

- Review any previous studies, including ERCP.
- Ultrasound, computed tomography (CT), or magnetic resonance imaging (MRI) ± magnetic resonance cholangiopancreatography (MRCP) can help identify dilated ducts and/or the level of obstruction for consideration of a target.
- Evaluate size and the orientation of the left hepatic lobe.
- Consider asymmetric dilatation of the bile ducts (right vs left); it would be prudent for the intervention to occur on the more dilated side.
- Decompressed biliary ducts are difficult to visualize and preclude a US-guided approach.
- Evaluate adjacent structures, such as the colon, heart, stomach and lung.

- Evaluate the left lobe of the liver for lesions, such as tumors or cysts, that may lie within the expected needle trajectory.

Laboratory Analyses

Evaluation of the patient's laboratory values should focus on identifying coagulopathy and liver dysfunction.

- INR >1.4: Correct through usual practices (vitamin K for elective cases, fresh frozen plasma [FFP] in emergent/urgent cases).
- Platelet count <50,000/dL: Platelet transfusions
  - Effective platelet half-life ($\sim$90 minutes).
  - Transfuse as the patient enters the room and/or administer during the procedure.
- PTT >50 seconds:
  - Hold heparin and low-molecular-weight heparins preprocedure according to their pharmacokinetics.
- Serum creatinine
  - May be important in cases where contrast administration might be injected intravenously, specifically when the biliary system is decompressed. The use of US minimizes the amount of contrast needed.

Patient Preparation

- Good intravenous access should be established in advance of the procedure and the patient should be adequately hydrated.
- The patient should having nothing by mouth (NPO) several hours before the procedure ($\geq$4 hours for conscious sedation.
- Prophylactic antibiotics should be administered 8 hours before the procedure when possible, and then repeated at the initiation of the procedure. Although there is no consensus on exact antibiotic regimen, coverage for both gram negatives should be administered. Postprocedure regimen can be tailored based on the results of aspirate cultures.
- Antibiotics should be administered intravenously with common choices including 1 g ceftriaxone, 1.5 to 3.0 g ampicillin/sulbactam; 1 g cefotetan plus 4 g mezlocillin; 2 g ampicillin plus 1.5 mg/kg gentamicin; in penicillin/cephalosporin allergies, vancomycin or clindamycin and aminoglycoside can be used.
- Conscious sedation with monitoring of vital signs during and after the procedure is generally maintained and achievable with midazolam and fentanyl.

PROCEDURE
Equipment/Supplies

- A multiarray 4-MHz to 5-MHz US transducer with Doppler capabilities is ideal for differentiating bile ducts from blood vessels.
- Optional needle-guide bracket.
- A sterile transducer cover, chlorhexidine cleansing fluid, and a fenestrated drape are used to prepare the sterile field.
- A 21-gauge needle with 10 to 20 mL of 1% lidocaine is used as a local anesthetic.
- An 11 blade for dermatomy for needle access.
- 21-gauge (diamond tip) or 22- gauge Chiba needle are needed for access. Use of a short needle is preferred for left-sided access given the short area to traverse.
- Syringe and flexible tube connector for injection of dilute contrast.
- An 0.018-inch wire for passage into the biliary system, either a stainless steel, nitinol, or hydrophilic-coated wire.
- For placement of the PBD
  - A 0.035-inch conversion system with a graduate dilation system with metal stiffener (eg, Neph-Set or Accustick; Boston Scientific, Natick, MA, USA).
  - Flexible 0.35 wire (Bentson and/or Glide wire) and a stiff 0.35 wire, such as an Amplatz.
  - 4-French or 5-French catheter (eg, Kumpe)
  - Fascial dilators (up to 8F).
  - 10-French or 12-French pigtail drainage catheter.

Preprocedure Ultrasound

- Visualize and evaluate the path to the target: a peripherally located, dilated, left intrahepatic bile duct. Doppler should be used to differentiate the bile ducts from blood vessels. In rare cases, a thrombosed blood vessel can mimic a bile duct. Motion of the bile ducts during the respiratory cycle and positioning with breath holding should also be assessed.
- The ideal skin entry site is just lateral to the xiphoid, approximately 2 cm from the subcostal margin, with avoidance of the rib cage. The skin site should be marked with the entry point corresponding to the needle-guide bracket. After marking, precise triangulation from the skin site to the bile ducts should be ascertained with US. Traditionally, the transducer orientation is transverse to the patient's abdomen/spine. Panning

toward the xiphoid can also be helpful. The angle achieved at the target duct should facilitate a wire passing from lateral to medial in the left biliary system, allowing for internalization of the biliary drain if the need arises.

Passage of Needle into Duct

- A 3-mm-deep incision is made with the scalpel, the 21-gauge or 22-gauge needle is inserted into the needle-guide bracket.
- The needle with stylet is directed toward, and inserted into the target bile duct without hesitation. US should visualize the needle within the duct.
- The stylet is removed and dilute contrast is injected (1:1 with saline or stronger) via a flexible connector and syringe.
- Fluoroscopic images should demonstrate needle placement within a peripheral bile duct, with the tip directed toward the common hepatic duct.
  - Very gentle contrast administration should be performed under maximum magnification. Overdistention of the ductal system can increase the risk for infection/sepsis.
  - Characteristic appearance of the biliary tree and a "dripping wax" appearance should be seen if successful in entry to the duct.
  - Brisk clearance indicates the needle is within a blood vessel. In this scenario, the needle may have passed through the bile duct target and should be carefully pulled back with continued gentle contrast injections in hopes of bile duct visualization.
  - If the needle enters a bile duct that is too central or with a poor angle for wire passage, this access can be used to opacify the ductal system with contrast material before abandoning. This will guide a second fluoroscopic at a better target. Alternatively, a second attempt at US access can be performed.

Access in the Biliary Tree with 0.018-inch Wire

Once the needle is in the appropriate duct, the 0.018-inch wire should be passed into the duct in consideration of further intervention or PBD. There are several variations in the method of achieving this aim and vary with type of wire used.

- *Significantly dilated ducts*: Operator places a gentle guiding curve on an *0.018-inch stainless steel or nitinol wire* and loads into

the needle in a tip-to-tip fashion. Slight retraction of the needle causes the preformed wire to "flop" into place and thus navigated along the duct. The retracted needle, outside the bile duct, provides support as the wire is advanced more centrally (**Fig. 1**).
- *Challenging biliary anatomy (eg, transplant, cholangitis, strictures)*: use of an *0.018-inch hydrophilic wire* may be helpful. This technique relies on passing through both sides of the duct and probing gently with the wire as the needle is retracted. Visual and haptic feedback guides the operator as to appropriate entry of the wire into the duct. Care should be given to advancing this wire, as dissection along the portal triad is possible. Resistance or coiling of the wire should be minimal; coiling may cause the wire to jam and both needle and wire will have to be retracted, abandoning the access attempt.

Biliary Drain Placement/Intervention

- After the 0.018-inch wire is advanced centrally within the appropriate duct, the needle is removed and a coaxial conversion system is used (eg, Accustick set) to upsize to a 0.035-inch (or 0.038-inch) wire.
- Exchange for a 0.035-inch guide wire is performed (eg, Bentson or Glide).
- A 4-French catheter (eg, Kumpe) working over the 0.035-inch guide wire can then be used to achieve central access into the

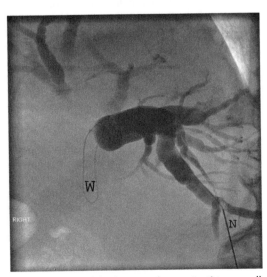

Fig. 1. Fluoroscopic image demonstrating needle access (N) of a dilated left intrahepatic bile duct. The wire (W) is directed toward the common hepatic duct.

small bowel in most cases (**Figs. 2** and **3**). If a central obstruction prohibits easy passage, a sheath might be considered to maintain access.

- Once the wire is in the small bowel (or to the central obstruction), a stiffer wire, such as an Amplatz wire, is placed through the catheter. The catheter is removed and wire access maintained.
  ○ In some instances, at this point stenting at the obstruction could be performed if desired clinically, providing palliative internal drainage. Resection candidates generally should not be stented.
- For PBD, once the 0.035-inch wire is in place, serial dilation is performed with fascial dilators, to an appropriate dilation for either a 10-French or 12-French biliary drain.

Drain Selection

- If the obstruction could not be passed, a strict *external drainage* will be required.
- *Internal-external drainage* catheters allow drainage both into the external bag and into the bowel via sideholes above and below the obstruction. Additional side holes can be cut if needed to ensure holes are both above and below the obstruction, providing adequate drainage.
- A *"pullback cholangiogram"* may be necessary to establish the level of obstruction. A guiding catheter or long sheath advanced over the wire allows passage of a second parallel wire. Leaving the safety wire in place, injection of contrast through the

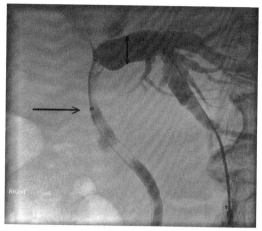

Fig. 3. Fluoroscopic image demonstrating introduction of the catheter (*arrow*) with passage along the wire into the left intrahepatic and common hepatic ducts. The 2-way arrow demonstrates dilatation of the left intrahepatic bile ducts.

side arm of the sheath (or into the guiding catheter) is performed as it is retracted.

- Postprocedural imaging should document the pigtail drain terminating within the small bowel (**Fig. 4**).
- Filling defects within the biliary system are likely a result of clotted blood, and should raise clinical suspicion for hemobilia.
- The pigtail drain should be left to gravity drainage and secured to the skin. A single silk suture and Percufix or Molnar disk generally provide adequate security against inadvertent dislodgement.

MANAGEMENT

For diagnostic PTC, success is determined by visualization of the opacified biliary tract. For

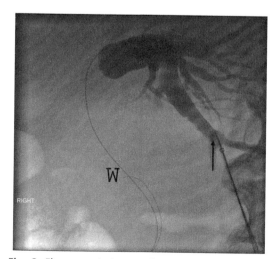

Fig. 2. Fluoroscopic image demonstrating introduction of the catheter (*arrow*) with passage along the wire into the left intrahepatic and common hepatic ducts.

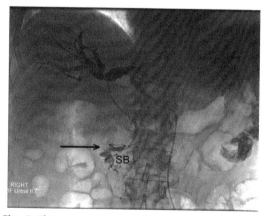

Fig. 4. Fluoroscopic images demonstrating successful placement of the drain, with pigtail component (*arrow*) coiling in the small bowel (SB).

PBD, success is marked by contrast from the pigtail portion of catheter in the small bowel. Technical success or failure is in large part determined by the degree of ductal dilatation. In a decompressed biliary ductal system, success rates can be as low as 40% for drainage placement and 65% for diagnostic PTCs.

Postprocedure Care

- Hospital admission is standard.
  - For a diagnostic PTC, the patient can be admitted for a 23-hour observation status.
  - For PBD, the drain output should be monitored for 24 to 48 hours with gravity drainage.
- After 4 hours of bed rest, activity can generally be advanced as tolerated.
- Advance diet as tolerated.
- Monitor blood pressure, heart rate, and oxygen saturation for signs of hemothorax or pneumothorax. Obtain chest x-ray if appropriate.
- Discontinue antibiotics after 24 hours if no signs of infection.
- Drain maintenance:
  - Monitor character and quantity of output.
  - A small amount of blood-tinged fluid postprocedurally is a common finding, which should clear with time.
  - If drain output is minimal, the drain should be flushed with 5 to 7 mL of sterile saline owing to decreased the viscosity of the bile.
  - Drainage up to 500 to 800 mL in 24 hours is not unusual.
  - For an internal-external drain, an overnight (~8 hour) capping trial should be performed. The patient can be discharged safely only after a capping trial with the absence of pain or fever.
  - If patient is discharged with tube capped, he or she should be given clear instructions to watch for fever and/or pain and to monitor drainage from the bag.

Hypovolemia

Electrolyte and fluid loss from the procedure can be substantial; thus, intravenous fluid hydration, ideally with lactated Ringer's solution to replace potassium, helps to alleviate these losses. A clear liquid diet can be started immediately and advanced as tolerated, often helping to alleviate the patient's nausea and vomiting.

Pain

Pain control with oral narcotics, such as acetaminophen and hydrocodone, can be administered after drainage. Careful clinical assessment of the patient's pain, laboratory values (specifically hematocrit), and the patient's vital signs (hypotension and increased heart rate) should be monitored for signs and symptoms of hypovolemia. If there is suspicion for hemorrhage, a regional US or noncontrast CT examination of the abdomen can be performed.

Bleeding

Postprocedural bleeding can occur from different etiologies, and imaging should assess for hemobilia, subcapsular hematoma, and hemothorax. First and foremost, a physical examination should assess for bleeding at the skin site. Management should include prompt capping of the tube in an effort to tamponade the bleed. In the setting of suspected bleeding, aggressive resuscitation with crystalline fluid boluses should be commenced. The patient should be typed and crossed, with blood transfusion occurring with hematocrits less than 30%.

Angiography can be helpful if there is suspicion of a portal venous or hepatic arterial bleed. A hepatic tract sinogram with subsequent upsizing of the tract can potentially tamponade a portal venous bleed. A hepatic angiogram can identify an arterial bleed, in which case selective arterial embolization can be performed. In cases of continued, unidentified bleeding, global gelfoam embolization can be considered, but is contraindicated in cases of severe liver dysfunction. A surgical consult should be obtained in cases of continued unidentified bleeding.

Bowel Perforation

Surgical consultation should also be obtained in the unlikely setting where the drain perforates a segment of bowel. The patient should be monitored for signs and symptoms of an acute abdomen, in which case the patient should be taken immediately to surgery. Otherwise, the tube should be left in place, allowing for the formation of a fistula, in which case the procedure can be performed in an elective setting.

Infection

Cholangitis occurs in approximately 3% of cases. In rare cases, this can lead to life-threatening biliary sepsis. Prophylactic antibiotics as mentioned previously should be administered preprocedurally in all cases, and continued if sepsis is suspected. Prompt transfer to the intensive care unit along with aggressive fluid resuscitation should occur in cases of suspected sepsis. If following a PTC, placement of a PBD should be performed immediately.

FURTHER READINGS

Citron SJ, Martin LG. Benign biliary strictures: treatment with percutaneous cholangioplasty. Radiology 1991;178:339–41.

Covey A, Brown K. Percutaneous transhepatic biliary drainage. Tech Vasc Interv Radiol 2008;11:14–20.

Dogra V, Saad WE. Ultrasound-guided procedures. Thieme Medical Publishers; 2009.

Lee MJ, Mueller PR, Saini S, et al. Percutaneous dilatation of benign biliary strictures: single-session therapy with general anesthesia. AJR Am J Roentgenol 1991;157:1263–6.

Mueller PR, Harbin WP, Ferrucci JT, et al. Fine-needle transhepatic cholangiography: reflections after 450 cases. AJR Am J Roentgenol 1981;136:85–90.

Mueller PR, vanSonnenberg E, Ferrucci JT, et al. Biliary stricture dilatation: multicenter review of clinical management in 73 patients. Radiology 1986;160:17–22.

Pomerantz B. Biliary tract interventions. Tech Vasc Interv Radiol 2009;12:162–70.

Saad WE, Davies MG, Darcy M. Management of bleeding after percutaneous cholangiography or transhepatic biliary drain placement. Tech Vasc Interv Radiol 2008;11:60–71.

Saad WE. Transhepatic techniques for accessing the biliary tract. Tech Vasc Interv Radiol 2008;11:21–42.

Saad WE, Wallace MJ, Wojak JC, et al, Journal of Interventional Radiology Standards of Practice Committee. Quality improvement guidelines for percutaneous transhepatic cholangiography and biliary drainage. J Vasc Interv Radiol 2010;21:789–95.

Venkatesan A, Kundu S, Sacks D, et al. Practice guideline for adult antibiotic prophylaxis during vascular and interventional radiology procedures. J Vasc Interv Radiol 2010;21:1611–20.

PERCUTANEOUS CHOLECYSTOSTOMY
Introduction

Acute cholecystitis is a common condition with the preferred treatment consisting of cholecystectomy along with prophylactic antibiotics. In young otherwise healthy patients, mortality is low, at approximately 1%. In older patients with comorbid conditions, however, mortality can be as high as 30%. In these patients, cholecystectomy is often contraindicated because of the patient's acute or chronic comorbidities. Percutaneous cholecystostomy offers a minimally invasive method to treat acute cholecystitis in this patient population. This part of the article focuses primarily on US-guided percutaneous gallbladder access.

Indications

- Drainage of an infected gallbladder in a critically ill patient, specifically a poor surgical candidate for cholecystectomy.
- As a temporary measure, offering a bridge to future definitive cholecystectomy.
- Access for other interventions, such as the removal/lithotripsy of a biliary stone.
- Visualization and drainage of the biliary ducts, in cases with a patent cystic duct.

Contraindications

As with biliary interventions, there are no absolute but relative contraindications relate to uncorrected coagulopathy and large-volume ascites.

- Uncorrected coagualopathy
  - INR: >1.4
  - Platelets: <50,000 to 70,000
  - PTT: >50 seconds. The clinician must take efforts to correct the coagulopathy, and must weigh this factor against the degree of clinical urgency to determine relative versus absolute contraindications.
- A gallbladder completely filled with stones or entirely decompressed, as well as a porcelain gallbladder, can prevent successful placement of the drainage catheter.

Risks

The overall major complication rate for percutaneous cholecystostomy is on the order of 3% to 8% (with 18-gauge or smaller needles).

The primary risks related to percutaneous cholecystostomy are:

- Hemorrhage (life threatening with injury to the cystic artery)
- Infection
  - Biliary sepsis or peritonitis (life threatening)
  - Cholangitis, abscess formation
- Bile leak/gallbladder perforation
- Pneumothorax.

Bleeding is most often transient; however, in rare cases can result in the need for blood transfusion, hepatic arterial embolization, or surgery. Risk depends on the patient's clinical scenario, as these patients are critically ill, with malignancy, cholangitis, and coagulopathy engendering increased risk.

Planning

Imaging

- Reviewing any previous studies, including US, CT, or MRI ± MRCP, can help to identify signs of acute cholecystitis: pericholecystic fluid, adjacent hepatic inflammation, and gallbladder wall thickening (**Figs. 5** and **6**).
- Hepatobiliary nuclear scan can offer a functional test to assess for acute cholecystitis.
- If cross-sectional imaging is available, multiplanar reformatted images can be used to visualize the angle of the needle, and demonstrate either a transperitoneal and/or transhepatic window for access.
- Evaluate adjacent structures, such as the colon, heart, stomach, and lung.
- A transhepatic approach should be considered, if these adjacent organs cannot be safely avoided.
- Evaluate the left lobe of the liver for lesions, such as tumors or cysts, that may lie within the expected needle trajectory.

Transhepatic versus transperitoneal approach

Transhepatic

- Theoretically lower chance of bile leak as needle enters the gallbladder through the extraperitoneal/bare area.
- The liver and gallbladder move together with respiration; thus, the needle is stabilized through the hepatic approach.

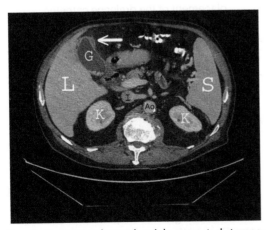

Fig. 5. Contrast-enhanced axial computed tomography image through the liver demonstrate thickening of the gallbladder wall (*arrow*) and pericholecystic stranding and adjacent hepatic inflammation. Ao, aorta; I, inferior vena cava; K, kidneys; L, Liver; G, gallbladder; S, spleen.

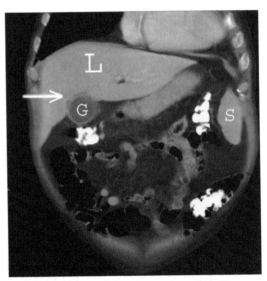

Fig. 6. Contrast-enhanced coronal computed tomography image through the liver demonstrate thickening of the gallbladder wall (*arrow*) and pericholecystic stranding and adjacent hepatic inflammation. L, Liver; G, gallbladder; S, spleen.

- Quicker maturation of the tract with a transhepatic approach.

Transperitoneal

- Useful in patients with hepatic lesions/tumors.
- Interposed bowel (Chialiditi syndrome) often makes the transhepatic approach not possible.
- Safer in cases of coagulopathy.
- May be required to obtain access along the long axis of the gallbladder for advanced interventions, such as stone extraction, and common bile duct access through the cystic duct.

Laboratory analyses

Evaluation of the patient's laboratory values should focus on identifying coagulopathy and liver dysfunction.

- INR >1.4: Correct through usual practices (vitamin K for elective cases, FFP in emergent/urgent cases).
- Platelet count <50,000/dL: Platelet transfusions
  - Effective platelet half-life (~90 minutes).
  - Transfuse as the patient enters the room and/or administer during the procedure.
- PTT >50 seconds:
  - Hold heparin and low-molecular-weight heparins before the procedure according to their pharmacokinetics.

Patient preparation

- Good intravenous access should be established in advance of the procedure and the patient should be adequately hydrated.
- The patient should be NPO several hours before the procedure ($\geq$4 h for conscious sedation).
- Prophylactic antibiotics should be administered 8 hours before the procedure when possible and then repeated at the initiation of the procedure. Although there is no consensus on exact antibiotic regimen, coverage for both gram negatives should be administered. Postprocedure regimen can be tailored based on the results of aspirate cultures.
- Antibiotics should be administered intravenously with common choices including 1 g ceftriaxone, 1.5 to 3.0 g ampicillin/sulbactam; 1 g cefotetan plus 4 g mezlocillin; 2 g ampicillin plus 1.5 mg/kg gentamicin; in penicillin/cephalosporin allergies, vancomycin or clindamycin and aminoglycoside can be used.
- Conscious sedation with monitoring of vital signs during and after the procedure is generally maintained and achievable with midazolam and fentanyl.

Procedure

Equipment/supplies

- A multiarray 4-MHz to 5-MHz US transducer with Doppler capabilities is ideal to localize blood vessels.
- Optional needle guide bracket.
- A sterile transducer cover, chlorhexidine cleansing fluid, and a fenestrated drape are used to prepare the sterile field.
- A 21-gauge needle with 10 to 20 mL of 1% lidocaine is used as a local anesthetic.
- An 11 blade for dermatomy for needle access.
- 18-gauge hypodermic (no stylet) needle is needed for access.
- Syringe and flexible tube connector for injection of dilute contrast.
- Flexible 0.35 wire (Bentson and/or Glide wire) and a stiff 0.35 wire such as an Amplatz.
  - 4-French or 5-French catheter (eg, Kumpe).
  - Fascial dilators (up to 8 French).
  - 10-French or 12-French pigtail drainage catheter.

Preprocedure US

- Visualize and evaluate the path to the target: specifically, the long axis of the gallbladder should be visualized (**Figs. 7** and **8**). Doppler can be used in transhepatic approaches to localize and avoid vessels.
- Motion of the gallbladder and liver during respiration, as well as positioning with breath holding should also be assessed.
- The ideal skin entry site is 2 cm from the subcostal margin, with avoidance of the rib cage. The skin site should be marked, after which careful triangulation from the skin site to the gallbladder should be ascertained.

Passage of needle into the gallbladder

- Injection of 1% lidocaine along the expected needle tract, intradermal to the gallbladder wall.
- Once a 3-mm-deep incision is made with the scalpel, the 18-gauge needle is directed toward the gallbladder.
- This needle should be connected by flexible tubing to a 20-mL syringe, which is partially filled with contrast material.
- Counter suction on the syringe is performed as the needle tip approaches the gallbladder.
- As the needle tip is seen entering the gallbladder, there should be simultaneous return of bile into the syringe. The needle should be positioned in the center of the gallbladder (**Fig. 9**).
- Once access has been achieved, fluoroscopy can be used to confirm that the needle tip is within the gallbladder.
- Fluoroscopic images should demonstrate needle placement within the center of the gallbladder.
  - Very gentle contrast administration should be performed under maximum

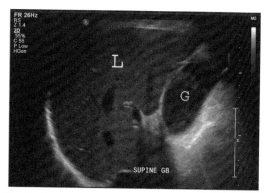

Fig. 7. Gray-scale image, transverse view of the gallbladder, which demonstrate a thickened wall and echogenic material, as well as shadowing stones within the gallbladder (G).

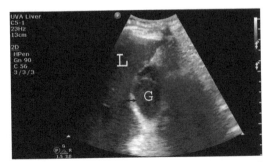

Fig. 8. Gray-scale image, sagittal view of the gallbladder, which demonstrate a thickened wall (*double arrow*) and echogenic material, as well as shadowing stones within the gallbladder (G).

magnification. Overdistention of the gallbladder can increase the risk for infection/sepsis.

○ Characteristic appearance of the gallbladder should be appreciated (**Fig. 10**). Compare with previous imaging in cases of filling defects, such as stones/sludge.

Gallbladder drain placement/intervention
- A 0.035-inch wire is advanced centrally through the needle and coiled within the gallbladder (**Fig. 11**), a 4-French catheter (eg, Kumpe) working over the 0.035-inch guide wire can then be used to achieve access in the gallbladder (**Fig. 12**).
- For percutaneous cholecystostomy, once the 0.035-inch wire is in place, serial dilation is performed with fascial dilators, to an appropriate dilation for either a 10-French or 12-French biliary drain.
- Careful attention should be taken to ensure that the dilator traverses the gallbladder wall, as opposed to pushing the wall distally along the wire.

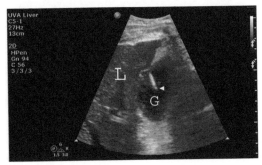

Fig. 9. Gray-scale image demonstrating the needle tip (*arrowhead*) appropriately positioned within the center of the gallbladder (G) during a percutaneous transhepatic cholecystostomy.

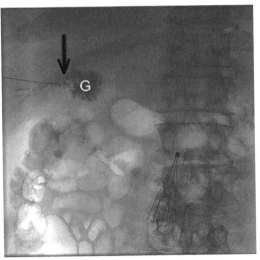

Fig. 10. Fluoroscopic image during a cholecystogram demonstrating the needle tip (*arrow*) entering the gallbladder (G), which is opacified with contrast and demonstrates internal debris.

Drainage placement
- Postprocedural imaging should document the pigtail drain terminating within the gallbladder (**Fig. 13**).
- New filling defects within the gallbladder are likely a result of clotted blood, and should raise clinical suspicion for hemorrhage.
- The pigtail drain should be left to gravity drainage and secured to the skin. A single silk suture and Percufix or Molnar disk generally provide adequate security against inadvertent dislodgement.

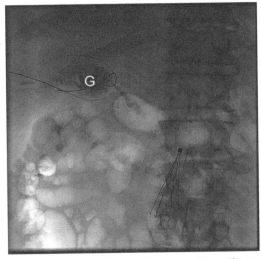

Fig. 11. Fluoroscopic image demonstrating coiling of the wire within the body of the gallbladder (G).

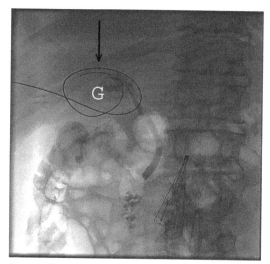

Fig. 12. Fluoroscopic image demonstrating the catheter (*arrow*) entering the gallbladder (G) over the wire.

Management

For percutaneous cholecystostomy, success is determined by visualization of the looped pigtail catheter within the gallbladder. Technical failure occurs in approximately 5% cases, and can be because of a decompressed gallbladder, significant cholelithiasis, porcelain gallbladder, or significant wall thickening. Clinical success is highly dependent on the patient's comorbidities and the role cholecystitis is playing in the patient's acute condition; thus, clinical success can vary from 60% to 90%.

Postprocedure care

- This procedure is performed exclusively on inpatients, many of whom are critically ill.

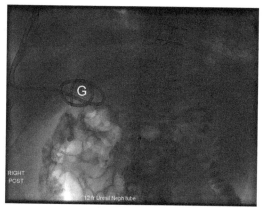

Fig. 13. Fluoroscopic image demonstrating the cholecystostomy drainage tube coiled appropriately in the gallbladder (G).

- Often activity is limited to bed rest.
- In floor patients without comorbid conditions, after 4 hours of bed rest, activity can be advanced as tolerated.
- Advance diet as tolerated.
- Monitor blood pressure, heart rate and oxygen saturation for signs of hemothorax or pneumothorax. Obtain chest x-ray if appropriate.
- After the procedure, the patient should be closely monitored for signs and symptoms of peritonitis or sepsis. Prompt transfer to the intensive care unit should occur if sepsis is suspected.
- Antibiotics often need to be continued for periods longer than 24 hours.
- Drain maintenance:
  - Monitor character and quantity of output.
  - A small amount of blood-tinged fluid postprocedurally is a common finding, which should clear with time.
  - If there is suspicion of blockage or tube displacement, the drain should be flushed with 5 to 7 mL of sterile saline owing to decreased the viscosity of the bile. This is generally performed after a contrasted fluoroscopic examination of the tube.
  - Contrast exams should otherwise be limited to 48 hours after the procedure because of biliary-portal reflux.
  - Drainage up to 500 to 800 mL in 24 hours is not unusual.

Hypovolemia

Electrolyte and fluid loss from the procedure can be substantial; thus, aggressive intravenous fluid hydration, ideally with lactated Ringer's solution for potassium replacement, especially over the first 24 hours, helps to alleviate these losses. The patient's diet can be advanced as tolerated; however, this is often not plausible given the patient's underlying medical illnesses.

Pain

The patient's pain level should be closely monitored, and narcotics are often required, specifically in the setting of peritonitis. Careful clinical assessment of the patient's pain, laboratory values (specifically hematocrit), and the patient's vital signs (hypotension and increased heart rate) should be monitored for signs and symptoms of hypovolemia. If there is suspicion for hemorrhage, a regional US or noncontrast CT examination of the abdomen can be performed.

Bleeding

Postprocedural bleeding can occur from different etiologies, and imaging should assess for hemobilia, subcapsular hematoma, and hemo-thorax. First and foremost, a physical examination should assess for bleeding at the skin site. In the setting of suspected bleeding, aggressive resuscitation with crystalline fluid boluses should be commenced. The patient should be typed and crossed, with blood transfusion occurring with hematocrits less than 30%.

Angiography can be helpful if there is suspicion of a hepatic arterial bleed. A hepatic angiogram can identify an arterial bleed, in which case selective arterial embolization can be performed. In cases of continued, unidentified bleeding, global gelfoam embolization can be considered, but is contraindicated in cases of severe liver dysfunction. A surgical consult should be obtained in cases of continued unidentified bleeding.

Bowel perforation

Surgical consultation should also be obtained in the unlikely setting where the drain perforates a segment of bowel. The patient should be monitored for signs and symptoms of an acute abdomen, in which case the patient should be taken immediately to surgery. Otherwise, the tube should be left in place, allowing for the formation of a fistula, in which case the procedure can be performed in an elective setting.

Infection

Prophylactic antibiotics, as mentioned previously, should be administered preprocedurally in all cases, and continued if sepsis is suspected. Prompt transfer to the intensive care unit along with aggressive fluid resuscitation with possible vasopressors should occur in cases of suspected sepsis.

FURTHER READINGS

Akhan O, Akinci D, Ozmen MN. Percutaneous cholecystostomy. Eur J Radiol 2002;43(3):229–36.

Chopra S, Dodd GD, Mumbower AL. Treatment of acute cholecystitis in non-critically ill patients at high surgical risk: comparison of clinical outcomes after gallbladder aspiration and after percutaneous cholecystostomy. AJR Am J Roentgenol 2000;176:1025–31.

Citron SJ, Martin LG. Benign biliary strictures: treatment with percutaneous cholangioplasty. Radiology 1991;178:339–41.

Covey A, Brown K. Percutaneous transhepatic biliary drainage. Tech Vasc Interv Radiol 2008;14–20.

Davis CA, Landercasper J, Gundersen LH, et al. Effective use of percutaneous cholecystostomy in high-risk surgical patients: techniques, tube management, and results. Arch Surg 1999;134:727–32.

Dogra V, Saad WE. Ultrasound-guided procedures. Thieme; 2009.

Famulari C, Macri A, Galipo S, et al. The role of ultrasonographic percutaneous cholecystostomy in the treatment of acute cholecystitis. Hepatogastroenterology 1996;43:538–41.

Hadas-Halpern I, Patlas M, Knizhnik M, et al. Percutaneous cholecystostomy in the management of cholecystitis. Isr Med Assoc J 2003;5:170–1.

Hamy A, Visset J, Likholatnikov D, et al. Percutaneous cholecystostomy for acute cholecystitis in critically ill patients. Surgery 1997;121:398–401.

Hatjidakis AA, Karampekios S, Parassopoulos P, et al. Maturation of the tract after percutaneous cholecystostomy with regards to the access route. Cardiovasc Intervent Radiol 1998;21:36–40.

Hatjidakis AA, Parassopoulos P, Petinarakis P, et al. Acute cholecystitis in high-risk patients: percutaneous cholecystostomy vs. conservative treatment. Eur Radiol 2002;12:1778–84.

Ito K, Fujita N, Noda Y, et al. Percutaneous cholecystostomy versus gallbladder aspiration for acute cholecystitis: a prospective randomized controlled trial. AJR Am J Roentgenol 2004;183:193–6.

Lee MJ, Mueller PR, Saini S, et al. Percutaneous dilatation of benign biliary strictures: single-session therapy with general anesthesia. AJR Am J Roentgenol 1991;157:1263–6.

Lo LD, Vogelzang RL, Braun MA, et al. Percutaneous cholecystostomy for the diagnosis and treatment of acute calculous and acalculous cholecystitis. J Vasc Interv Radiol 1995;6:629–34.

Mueller PR, Harbin WP, Ferrucci JT, et al. Fine-needle transhepatic cholangiography: reflections after 450 cases. AJR Am J Roentgenol 1981;136:85–90.

Mueller PR, vanSonnenberg E, Ferrucci JT Jr, et al. Biliary stricture dilatation: multicenter review of clinical management in 73 patients. Radiology 1986;160:17–22.

Patel M, Miedema BW, James MA, et al. Percutaneous cholecystostomy is an effective treatment for high-risk patients with acute cholecystitis. Am Surg 2000;66:33–7.

Pomerantz BJ. Biliary tract interventions. Tech Vasc Interv Radiol 2009;12(2):162–70.

Saad WE, Davies MG, Darcy M. Management of bleeding after percutaneous cholangiograhy or transhepatic biliary drain placement. Tech Vasc Interv Radiol 2008;11:60–71.

Saad WE, Wallace MJ, Wojak JC, et al, Journal of Interventional Radiology Standards of Practice Committee. Quality improvement guidelines for percutaneous transhepatic cholangiography and biliary drainage. J Vasc Interv Radiol 2010;21(6):789–95.

Saad WE. Transhepatic techniques for accessing the biliary tract. Tech Vasc Interv Radiol 2008;11:21–42.

Teoh WM, Cade RJ, Banting SW, et al. Percutaneous cholecystostomy in the management of acute cholecystitis. Aust N Z J Surg 2005;75:396–8.

Venkatesan A, Kundu S, Sacks D, et al. Practice guideline for adult antibiotic prophylaxis during vascular and interventional radiology procedures. J Vasc Interv Radiol 2010;21(11):1611–20.

Welschbillig-Meunier K, Pessaux P, Lebigot J, et al. Percutaneous cholecystostomy for high-risk patients with acute cholecystitis. Surg Endosc 2005;19:1256–9.

Ultrasound-Guided Percutaneous Nephrostomy

Matthew R. Bernhard, MD[a],*, Allison J. Lippert, MD[a],
Minhaj S. Khaja, MD, MBA[a], Wael E. Saad, MBBCh, FSIR[b]

KEYWORDS

- Percutaneous nephrostomy • Ultrasound • Renal collecting system • Image-guided procedure

KEY POINTS

- Clinical evaluation and review of anatomic and functional imaging is essential in selecting appropriate candidates before percutaneous nephrostomy (PCN) to ensure technical and clinical success.
- Ultrasound-guided PCN is ideal when there is moderate dilatation of the renal collecting system.
- Needle access of the appropriate calyx should be to the tailored to the planned intervention, ranging from urinary diversion to nephrolithotomy.
- Postnephrostomy narcotics are not typically required. If pain persists, attention should be paid to underlying cause of the patient's disproportionate pain.
- Overall mortality for all indications of PCN is estimated at less than 0.1%.

INTRODUCTION

Percutaneous nephrostomy (PCN) is a procedure in which percutaneous access of the kidney is obtained to provide external drainage in an obstructed renal collecting system or serve as a conduit through which minimally invasive urologic procedures can be performed. Ultrasound-guided PCN has been validated as an effective and safe minimally invasive image-guided procedure. This article reviews the indications, preprocedural patient evaluation, techniques, postprocedural management, and complications of ultrasound-guided PCN.

INDICATIONS

The most common indications for PCN include (in descending order of incidence) decompression of an obstructed renal collecting system, providing access for minimally invasive urologic interventions, urinary diversion, and palliation of pain secondary to renal calculi or pregnancy.[1–5] Less commonly, urinary obstruction may be caused by retroperitoneal fibrosis or pelvic masses, such as cervical and endometrial carcinoma, prostate cancer, bladder cancer, lymphoma, and other soft tissue or stromal malignancies.

Decompression of an obstructed renal collecting system is performed to improve renal function in the setting of benign or malignant urinary obstruction, including the treatment of pyonephrosis. An infected, obstructed urinary system is an urgent indication for PCN. Urinary tract obstruction with impairment of renal function is an urgent rather than an emergent indication, with renal transplants being the exception because of their tenuous nature. Hydronephrosis is not synonymous with urinary obstruction, and therefore is not an indication for PCN. Hydronephrosis may be present for months after decompression of the obstructed collecting system. Acute high-grade urinary obstruction induces anuria; thus, acute obstruction does not result in the distention

[a] Division of Vascular and Interventional Radiology, Radiology and Medical Imaging, University of Virginia Health System, Charlottesville, VA, USA; [b] Division of Vascular Interventional Radiology, Department of Radiology and Imaging Sciences, University of Virginia Health System, Charlottesville, VA, USA
* Corresponding author.
E-mail address: mattbernhard@virginia.edu

Ultrasound Clin 7 (2012) 413–420
doi:10.1016/j.cult.2012.03.005
1556-858X/12/$ – see front matter Published by Elsevier Inc.

of the collecting system. In addition, nonobstructive physiologic hydronephrosis has several causes, including postobstructive relief, pregnancy, polydipsia and polyuria, diuretics, overhydration, and congenital causes.

As the breadth of minimally invasive urologic interventions continues to evolve, percutaneous access of the renal collecting system is increasing in importance. Subsequent minimally invasive urologic procedures include percutaneous nephrolithotomy (PCNL) and ureteral interventions, such as balloon dilation and stent placement of ureteral strictures, embolization of ureteric fistulas, biopsy, or traversing a transected ureter in the setting of trauma.

PREPROCEDURAL EVALUATION

Preprocedural evaluation of the patient is essential before PCN. Proper evaluation includes review of available cross-sectional and functional imaging and laboratory data. The technical success of the procedure requires a detailed evaluation of the location, orientation, and anatomy of the target kidney. Orientation should be analyzed for any rotational abnormality that may affect the axis of the kidney. In severe cases of malrotation and/or malposition of the kidney, a transabdominal approach may be required in place of the standard transretroperitoneal approach. Preprocedural knowledge of the location and orientation of the kidney aids in planning patient positioning, decreases time gaining access, and reduces complications.

A detailed evaluation of the anatomy of the target kidney for variant anatomic and structural renal abnormality helps determine the desired access site. Special attention should be paid to the presence or absence of a duplicated renal collecting system. If a duplicated system is present, the extent of the duplication and which moiety is affected are essential to determine. Accessing the wrong moiety subjects the patient to an additional unnecessary procedure and the associated potential complications.

Careful attention should be given to underlying structural renal abnormality that can impact preprocedural planning, such as renal cysts, calyceal diverticula, tumors, and calculi. Renal cysts and calyceal diverticula should be identified to avoid inadvertent access, which would prevent drainage or access of the renal collecting system. Renal tumors are typically hypervascular and would therefore have a high propensity to bleed if traversed. Passing a PCN drain through a renal tumor also may increase the risk of tumor dissemination along the catheter tract.

Nephrolithiasis can be both beneficial and detrimental, depending on the size and location of the stones.[6] Calculi can be used as fluoroscopic landmarks if ultrasound-guided access of the collecting system is difficult. In addition, calyces completely occupied by a single calculus may hinder the needle from passing through the infundibulum to the renal pelvis. Finally, the presence of residual contrast should be noted. A delayed nephrogram or pyelogram can be used as a fluoroscopic landmark if the operator has difficulty accessing the collecting system with ultrasound. Structural abnormalities may be incidental to the indications for the procedure and should therefore not be overlooked.

Assessment of the paranephric anatomy is crucial for planning PCN.[7,8] Preprocedural planning of the needle trajectory can reduce the likelihood of transgression of adjacent organs, decreasing the risk of potentially major complications. Organs of particular concern are the colon, spleen, and liver for native kidneys and small bowel for transplant kidneys.[1]

Preprocedural evaluation of dynamic functional imaging, in addition to static cross-sectional imaging, can help elucidate whether the origin and chronicity of the underlying abnormality necessitates PCN.[9] In cases of hydronephrosis identified with cross-sectional imaging, in the absence of diminished renal function, a nuclear renal scan can be used to determine whether renal obstruction is present. If a nuclear renal scan shows poor renal function in the absence of obstruction, PCN would not be indicated. Furthermore, a nuclear renal scan can identify the least functioning and/or most obstructed kidney in the setting of staging bilateral nephrostomy tubes.

Careful evaluation of laboratory values is an important preprocedural consideration in addition to clinical examination and cross-sectional imaging. The sole contraindication to PCN is uncorrected coagulopathy.[10–12] Whether coagulopathy is a relative or absolute contraindication depends on the degree of coagulopathy, the clinical setting, and the degree of urgency of PCN. A platelet count of greater than 50,000 to 70,000/mm^3 and an international normalized ratio less than 1.4 to 1.7 are commonly used guidelines followed by many institutions. These parameters have not been validated specifically, but rather represent a reflection of commonly used guidelines and operator comfort levels. Ultimately, the operator must consider the risks and benefits of the procedure.

Review of pretreatment serum creatinine is important to establish baseline renal function, which allows improvement of renal function to be assessed after nephrostomy tube placement. Furthermore, elevated serum creatinine identifies patients in whom intravenous contrast administration for anatomic definition would be contraindicated.

TECHNIQUES

Like most minimally invasive image-guided procedures, appropriate preprocedural preparation for PCN includes intravenous access, nothing-by-mouth (NPO) status for 6 to 8 hours before the procedure, planning images, and sterile technique. Adequate intravenous access is necessary for administration of moderate conscious sedation, fluid resuscitation, and prophylactic antibiotics, such as ciprofloxacin. With moderate sedation, most patients tolerate the procedure, and general anesthesia is not typically required.

After the patient is positioned prone or oblique prone on the fluoroscopy table, ultrasound imaging of the target kidney helps assess its anatomy and location. Ultrasound with a multiarray 4- to 5-MHz transducer is typically used to determine the easiest approach to the target calyx, assess renal mobility during breathing and breath-holds, assess retroperitoneal anatomy, and triangulate the target calyx (usually the lower pole calyx) with the appropriate skin access site. Manipulation of the transducer (with the attached bracketed needle guide) in a longitudinal orientation to the axis of the target kidney is the most commonly used approach; however, axial and oblique orientations may be necessary to appropriately determine the trajectory to access the desired calyx, preferably a dilated lower pole calyx. Maintaining a needle trajectory of 20° to 22° from midline at a distance spanning four fingerbreadths from the spinous processes below the level of T11 helps minimize complications. Maintaining the appropriate needle trajectory of 20° to 22° allows the needle to traverse the plane between the ventral two-thirds and dorsal one-third of the kidney, thereby reducing bleeding complications. This avascular plane created by the division of the main renal artery into ventral and dorsal branches is known as *the Brodel bloodless line of incision*. Using a distance greater than four fingerbreadths from the spinous processes helps approximate the region that passes between the back musculature and retroperitoneal viscera. If the access site is too medial, the nephrostomy drain will traverse skeletal muscle, including the psoas, which may result in increased pain, bleeding, and diminished drain function. If the access site is positioned too far lateral, the risk of colonic transgression and splenic laceration increases. When planning PCNL, the trajectory and angulations must be taken in to account to allow the urologist to maneuver from the proposed calyceal access to the renal calculi.

Needle Access of the Renal Collecting System

Needle access for PCN is primarily obtained through ultrasound guidance, fluoroscopy, or a combination of both.[13,14] CT-guided needle access is typically reserved for when all other guidance modalities have failed.[15] Different approaches to PCN include single-step ultrasound-guided definitive needle access, two-step access using ultrasound-guided access of the renal pelvis followed by definitive fluoroscopic needle access, or two-step access using fluoroscopy for access of the renal pelvis followed by needle access. Two-step access using fluoroscopic access of the renal pelvis followed by definitive fluoroscopic needle access is beyond the scope of this article. Each approach has inherent pros and cons, depending on operator experience and comfort with the different imaging modalities. No statistically significant difference exists between the various approaches in the setting of a nondilated renal pelvis.[16] In the setting of PCNL, ultrasound guidance is more efficacious, and possibly safer, than fluoroscopic guidance.[17,18]

Despite the choice of modality and approach, all patients are prepped and draped with a fenestrated drape, in accordance with standard surgical sterile technique. Using a 21-gauge needle, 1% lidocaine is administered at the planned access site. Deep infiltration is not necessary because of the insensitivity of the renal capsule (relative to the liver capsule), increasing the risk for potential complications without clear benefit.

Single-step ultrasound-guided needle access is ideally used in the presence of moderate dilatation of the renal collecting system (**Fig. 1**). Once adequate local analgesia is achieved, an incision is made using an 11-blade scalpel. The target calyx is then visualized with the ultrasound probe. An 18- to 22-gauge coaxial diamond-tip access needle is passed through the ultrasound needle guide bracket into the target calyx using a single firm pass. Slow or intermittent passage of the needle allows time for inadvertent repositioning of the ultrasound probe, potentially causing the needle to deflect off target. The ultrasound probe should be held still to maintain visibility of the needle tip and the target calyx at all times. If the full free length of the needle is introduced and calyceal access is not obtained, the needle attached to the transducer guide bracket can be dismantled, allowing for an additional 3 to 4 cm of needle depth.

Large caliber needles are preferred because of their increased stiffness and versatility. The stiffness of larger caliber needles affords a straighter path toward the target calyx. Additionally, 18- to 19-gauge needles accept the 0.035-in wire system

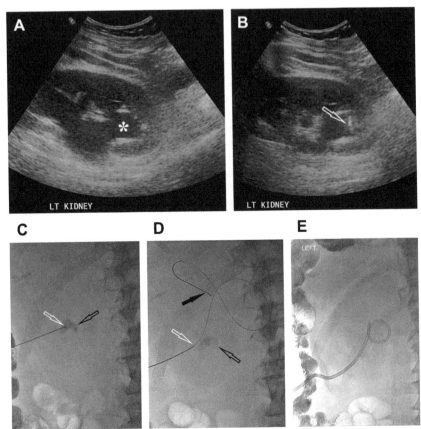

Fig. 1. (*A*) Longitudinal ultrasound image of the left kidney of a 75-year-old woman with new hydronephrosis. The renal pelvis is identified and targeted for needle placement by ultrasound (*asterisk*). (*B*) Ultrasound image showing the needle tip (*hollow arrow*) in the renal pelvis of the target kidney. (*C*) Fluoroscopic image showing the needle tip (*hollow white arrow*) in the contrast-opacified inferior pole calyx (*hollow black arrow*), confirming appropriate positioning. (*D*) Fluoroscopic image showing the guidewire (*solid black arrow*) coiled within a markedly dilated renal pelvis. (*E*) Fluoroscopic image showing the nephrostomy drainage-catheter within the unopacified left renal pelvis.

used for tract dilators and nephrostomy tubes. Smaller needles accept the 0.018-in wire system, necessitating the need for telescoped access to upsize to an 0.035- or 0.038-in platform. Alternatively, a trocar system can be used gain access under ultrasound guidance.[19]

Some operators may use a two-step needle access approach in which the renal pelvis is accessed with ultrasound guidance followed by contrast injection (with or without air) and definitive needle access using fluoroscopy. This technique is less commonly used than the single-step ultrasound-guided approach detailed earlier. This hybrid approach is currently reserved for when little or no calyceal dilatation is present or when intravenous contrast cannot be used to outline the renal collecting system (because of poor renal function or contrast allergy). A 21- or 22-gauge needle is used to access the renal pelvis using the single-pass method (detailed earlier) (**Fig. 2**A and B).

Contrast material can be introduced for better visualization of the renal pelvis before choosing the appropriate calyx (see **Fig. 2**C). Air can also be used, with the patient in the prone position to delineate the posterior calyces dependently filling with air (see **Fig. 2**D and E). Placement of definitive calyceal access is subsequently performed using a "second stick" under fluoroscopic guidance (see **Fig. 2**F and G).

Once the needle is in the desired position within the target calyx, the stylet is removed and the operator aspirates as the needle is slowly withdrawn. Return of urine confirms the presence of the needle tip within the collecting system.

Needle Placement Considerations

If access was obtained for general urinary diversion, needle placement in the posterior aspect of the lower pole calyx is preferred because this

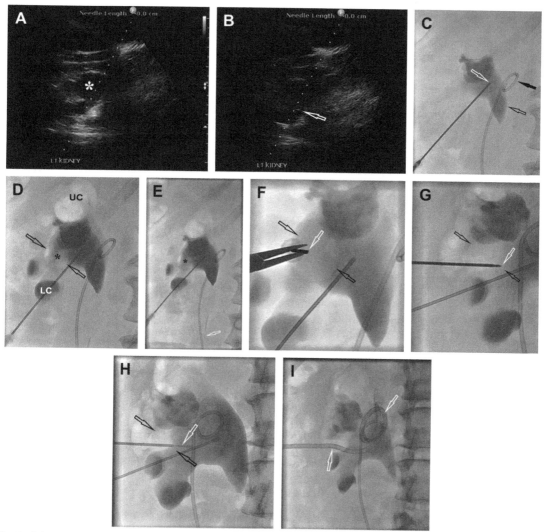

Fig. 2. (*A*) Longitudinal ultrasound image of the left kidney of a 60-year-old man with a history of nephrolithiasis. The renal pelvis is identified (*asterisk*) and targeted for needle placement by ultrasound. (*B*) Ultrasound image showing the needle tip (*hollow arrow*) in the renal pelvis of the target kidney. (*C*) Fluoroscopic image showing the needle tip (*hollow white arrow*) in the contrast-filled renal pelvis (*hollow black arrow*) of the target kidney. A ureteric stent outside the renal collecting system is noted incidentally (*solid arrow*). (*D*) Fluoroscopic image after injection of air into the renal pelvis to visualize the posterior calyces. Air layers dependently within the posterior calyces with the patient in the prone position. The image shows an air-filled middle-to-lower calyx (between *hollow arrows* and centered by the *asterisk*). The upper pole calyces (UC) are also filled with air. The lower calyx (LC) is filled with contrast. (*E*) Fluoroscopic image (from above) after injection of air shows a middle-to-lower calyx filled with air (*asterisk*). A radio-opaque ureteral calculus (*hollow arrow*) is identified in the proximal ureter. (*F*) Fluoroscopic image obtained as an 18-gauge needle (*hollow white arrow* at needle tip) is placed enface to the image intensifier (gunsite technique) over the air-filled target calyx (between *hollow black arrows*). (*G*) Oblique fluoroscopic image obtained as the 18-gauge needle (*hollow white arrow* at needle tip) is advanced into the air-filled target calyx (between *hollow black arrows*). The oblique image allows the operator to gauge needle depth. (*H*) Oblique fluoroscopic image obtained after contrast is injected through the 18-gauge needle. A jet of contrast is seen in the renal collecting system (*hollow white arrow*). The air-filled target calyx is again identified (between *hollow black arrows*). (*I*) Fluoroscopic image showing the nephrostomy drainage-catheter (*hollow arrows*) within the left renal pelvis.

minimizes risk of complications. However, if access is obtained to intervene on a renal calculus for PCNL, confirmation of the appropriate calyx is essential. Similarly, if access is obtained in anticipation of percutaneous ureteric interventions, the angle between the transperitoneal tract and the ureter through the renal collecting system must be taken into account. An angle that is too acute may hinder subsequent ureteric interventions. If the calyceal access is not ideal for the desired indication, several options are available using ultrasound, fluoroscopy, or a combination of the two. A simple alternative is to make a second attempt using ultrasound guidance once the first pass is removed.

Fluoroscopic-Guided Wire and Nephrostomy Tube Passage

After confirmation of the appropriate needle location for the desired indication, a formal antegrade diagnostic pyelogram may be performed to evaluate the collecting system (see **Fig. 2**H). The cause and level of the obstruction usually can be identified at this time. Urosepsis and pyuria are the major contraindications to pyelogram, because pressurizing the collecting system may cause or worsen sepsis. After the antegrade pyelogram, an 0.018- to 0.038-in access wire is then passed into the renal collecting system. Definitive needle access with a 21- to 22-gauge needle will accommodate an 0.018-in wire system, whereas access with an 18- to 19-gauge wire will accommodate an 0.035-in wire system. The 0.018-in wire system requires a composite access system (stiff, telescoped dilator) to upsize to a more rigid 0.035- or 0.038-in system. Once the 0.035-in guidewire is coiled in the renal pelvis, a skin incision is then made, tailored to the size of the planned access device. For example, an 8-French nephrostomy requires a 2- to 3-mm incision, whereas an 18- to 22-French device for PCNL requires a 6- to 7-mm incision. An 8-French fascial dilator is then passed to create a retroperitoneal tract. If larger devices are needed (eg, for PCNL), serial fascial dilations can be performed. Next, a nephrostomy tube (commonly 8- to 10-French) is advanced over the guidewire into the renal pelvis. Proper positioning should be confirmed before forming the pigtail. Once the distal loop is formed within the renal pelvis, the self-retaining string is locked and the tube is secured to the skin with sutures and placed to gravity drainage (see **Fig. 2**I). In patients with no evidence of overt infection or complications, a nephroureteral stent may be placed primarily, as opposed to a pigtail nephrostomy tube,

especially in patients with ureteral disease that can be easily traversed.

POSTNEPHROSTOMY EVALUATION AND MANAGEMENT
Postnephrostomy Imaging

Immediate postnephrostomy imaging is recommended to document appropriate placement of the pigtail end of nephrostomy tube within the renal pelvis. Visualization of contrast material around the collecting system or tracking along the ureter occurs with difficult nephrostomies in the setting of a decompressed collecting system or multiple initial needle passes. New filling defects within the collecting system are likely the result of clotted hematuria. Urine is frequently sanguineous, but frank blood should not be observed. Sanguineous urine that becomes bloodier over time is abnormal and requires further investigation. CT angiography (CTA) is the current standard for evaluating emergent PCN complications in the setting of hypotension or decreased hematocrit. CTA and Doppler ultrasound are helpful in evaluating arteriovenous fistulas or aneurysms. Conventional angiography can also be used, most commonly in the setting of known hemorrhage (documented by CTA) or when there is high clinical suspicion in the setting of negative or equivocal CTA.[20,21]

Postnephrostomy Observation

Although PCN is a minimally invasive procedure performed under conscious sedation, PCN should not be performed on an outpatient basis. The patient should be admitted for observation for a minimum of 23 hours. The patient should remain on bedrest for 4 to 6 hours. The patient's vital signs, hematocrit, and nephrostomy drain output should be closely monitored. Drainage of pus may require the drain to be flushed frequently to avoid blockage. After this period, the patient should be instructed on how to maneuver with the nephrostomy drains and be reminded that they are tethered to a collecting bag.

Pain Management

Narcotics are typically not required postnephrostomy. However, if pain persists at discharge, over-the-counter analgesics are usually sufficient. Occasionally, patients may require oral narcotic analgesics, such as oxycodone or hydrocodone. Intravenous narcotics can be prescribed in rare instances, but attention should be paid to underlying causes of the patient's disproportionate pain. If pain persists in the context of stable vital signs and hematocrit, renal ultrasound should be considered to evaluate for subcapsular hematoma. If pain persists in the setting of labile blood pressure or dropping hematocrit, however, a noncontrast CT or CTA should be performed to evaluate for retroperitoneal hematoma.

COMPLICATIONS AND THEIR MANAGEMENT

The major complications of PCN are bleeding, infection, and injury to the surrounding viscera.[1,20–23] Overall mortality for all indications of PCN is estimated at less than 0.1%.[9] Bleeding typically presents clinically as hematuria. Postnephrostomy frank hematuria not requiring transfusion is the most common bleeding complication, and can be managed by capping the drain to tamponade bleeding while further investigation of the cause is undertaken. Other bleeding complications, although less frequent, include subcapsular hematoma, extracapsular retroperitoneal hematoma, access-site bleeding, arteriovenous fistula, and hemothorax. Bleeding is typically transient, but if it is clinically significant, management should include volume resuscitation with crystalloid fluid and blood products, serial hematocrit measurements, and surgical consultation as necessary. In rare cases, transcatheter arterial embolization or exploratory surgery and nephrectomy may be required.[20,24–28]

Infection, including sepsis, occurs in 1% to 3% of all cases and 7% to 9% of pyonephrosis cases.[29,30] In cases of documented urinary tract infection, prophylactic antibiotics should be administered.[31,32] Caution should be taken to avoid overdistention of the collecting system with contrast material, minimizing the potential for transmigration of pathogens into the venous circulation. In the setting of postprocedural fever, intravenous antibiotics should be considered and urine and blood cultures should be obtained.

Injury to the surrounding viscera primarily concerns passage through bowel or pleura, resulting in pneumoperitoneum, pneumothorax, or hemothorax. Thoracic complications are rare and typically encountered during percutaneous access of the superior pole calyces for nephrolithotomies. Transgression of adjacent visceral organs is also rare, most commonly involving the spleen and colon in native kidneys and small bowel in renal transplants. If the drain traverses bowel, the drain should be left in place to allow a tract to mature. After the patient recovers from their acute condition, the drain should be removed to minimize the risk of development of a chronic nephrocolonic fistula.

SUMMARY

PCN has been proven to be an effective and safe minimally invasive image-guided procedure. The procedure provides great versatility as a method of external drainage of the renal collecting system and as a portal for an evolving variety of minimally invasive urologic interventions.

REFERENCES

1. Dyer RB, Regan JD, Kavanagh PV, et al. Percutaneous nephrostomy with extensions of the technique: step by step. Radiographics 2002;22:503–25.
2. Hausegger KA, Portugaller HR. Percutaneous nephrostomy and antegrade ureteral stenting: technique-indications-complications. Eur Radiol 2006;16: 2016–30.
3. Avritscher R, Madoff DC, Ramirez PT, et al. Fistulas of the lower urinary tract: percutaneous approaches for the management of a difficult clinical entity. Radiographics 2004;24:S217–36.
4. Adamo R, Saad WE, Brown DB. Percutaneous ureteral interventions. Tech Vasc Interv Radiol 2009;12(3):205–15.
5. Saad WE, Moorthy M, Ginat D. Percutaneous nephrostomy: native and transplanted kidneys. Tech Vasc Interv Radiol 2009;12(3):172–92.
6. Zagoria RJ, Dyer RB. Do's and don't's of percutaneous nephrostomy. Acad Radiol 1999;6:370–7.
7. Chalasani V, Bissoon D, Bhuvanagir AK, et al. Should PCNL patients have a CT in the prone position preoperatively? Can J Urol 2010;17(2):5082–6.
8. Tuttle DN, Yeh BM, Meng MV, et al. Risk of injury to adjacent organs with lower-pole fluoroscopically guided percutaneous nephrostomy: evaluation with prone, supine, and multiplanar reformatted CT. J Vasc Interv Radiol 2005;16(11):1489–92.
9. Thomsen HS, Hvid-Jacobsen K, Meyhoff HH, et al. Combination of DMSA-scintigraphy and hippuran renography in unilateral obstructive nephropathy. Improved prediction of recovery after intervention. Acta Radiol 1987;28(5):653–5.
10. Stables DP, Ginsberg NJ, Johnson ML. Percutaneous nephrostomy: a series and review of the literature. Am J Roentgenol 1978;130:75–82.
11. Farrell TA, Hicks ME. A review of radiologically guided percutaneous nephrostomies in 303 patients. J Vasc Interv Radiol 1997;8:769–74.
12. Bozkurt OF, Resorlu B, Yildiz Y, et al. Retrograde intrarenal surgery versus percutaneous nephrolithotomy in the management of lower-pole renal stones with a diameter of 15 to 20 mm. J Endourol 2011; 25(7):1131–5.
13. Mahmood T, Younus R, Ahmad F, et al. Ultrasound as a reliable guidance system for percutaneous nephrostomy. J Coll Physicians Surg Pak 2007;17:15–8.

14. Basiri A, Ziaee SA, Nasseh H, et al. Totally ultrasonography-guided percutaneous nephrolithotomy in the flank position. J Endourol 2008;22:1453–7.

15. Sommer CM, Huber J, Radeleff BA, et al. Combined CT- and fluoroscopy-guided nephrostomy in patients with non-obstructive uropathy due to urine leaks in cases of failed ultrasound-guided procedures. Eur J Radiol 2011;80(3):686–91.

16. Montvilas P, Solvig J, Johansen TE. Single-centre review of radiologically guided percutaneous nephrostomy using "mixed" technique: success and complication rates. Eur J Radiol 2011;80(2):553–8.

17. Basiri A, Ziaee AM, Kianian HR, et al. Ultrasonographic versus fluoroscopic access for percutaneous nephrolithotomy: a randomized clinical trial. J Endourol 2008;22:281–4.

18. Hosseini MM, Hassanpour A, Farzan R, et al. Ultrasonography-guided percutaneous nephrolithotomy. J Endourol 2009;23:603–7.

19. Newhouse JH, Pfister RC. Percutaneous catheterization of the kidney and perinephric space: trocar technique. Urol Radiol 1981;2:157–64.

20. Gupta S, Gulati M, Uday SK, et al. Percutaneous nephrostomy with real-time sonographic guidance. Acta Radiol 1997;38:454–7.

21. Radecka E, Magnusson A. Complications associated with percutaneous nephrostomies. A retrospective study. Acta Radiol 2004;45:184–8.

22. Vijay MK, Vijay P, Das RK, et al. Renal artery pseudoaneurysm following percutaneous nephrolithotomy. Saudi J Kidney Dis Transpl 2011;22(2):347–8.

23. Hopper KD, Yakes WF. The posterior intercostal approach for percutaneous renal procedures: risk of puncturing the lung, spleen, and liver as determined by CT. AJR Am J Roentgenol 1990;154:115–7.

24. Lee WJ, Mond DJ, Patel M, et al. Emergency percutaneous nephrostomy: technical success based on level of operator experience. J Vasc Interv Radiol 1994;5:327–30.

25. Harris RD, Walther PC. Renal arterial injury associated with percutaneous nephrostomy. Urology 1984;23:215–7.

26. Sadick M, Röhrl B, Schnülle P, et al. Multislice CT-angiography in percutaneous postinterventional hematuria and kidney bleeding: influence of diagnostic outcome on therapeutic patient management. Arch Med Res 2007;38(1):126–32.

27. Vignali C, Lonzi S, Bargellini I, et al. Vascular injuries after percutaneous renal procedures: treatment by transcatheter embolization. Eur Radiol 2004;14:723–9.

28. Yamaguchi A, Skolarikos A, Buchholz NP, et al. Operating times and bleeding complications in percutaneous nephrolithotomy: a comparison of tract dilation methods in 5,537 patients in the clinical research office of the endourological society percutaneous nephrolithotomy global study. J Endourol 2011;25(6):933–9.

29. Lewis S, Patel U. Major complications after percutaneous nephrostomy lessons from a department audit. Clin Radiol 2004;59:171–9.

30. Rao PN, Dube DA, Weightman NC, et al. Prediction of septicemia following endourological manipulation for stones in the upper urinary tract. J Urol 1991;146:955–60.

31. McDermott VG, Schuster MG, Smith TP. Antibiotic prophylaxis in vascular and interventional radiology. AJR Am J Roentgenol 1997;169:31–8.

32. Spies JB, Rosen RJ, Lebowitz AS. Antibiotic prophylaxis in vascular and interventional radiology: a rational approach. Radiology 1988;166:381–7.

Index

Note: Page numbers of article titles are in **boldface** type.

Ultrasound Clin 7 (2012) 421–424
doi:10.1016/S1556-858X(12)00053-9

Printed and bound by CPI Group (UK) Ltd, Croydon, CR0 4YY

03/10/2024

01040357-0020